ENDORSEMENTS

In this book, Dr. Tianne Foster provides a concise but comprehensive review of the major themes regarding job burnout: its causes and its impact. Her ideas for taking action convey a deep understanding of the underlying issues and the role of workplace leaders and clinicians in developing more fulfilling and sustainable workplaces.

— Michael P. Leiter, PhD
Michael Leiter & Associates
Professor Emeritus, Acadia University

Working as a pharmacist, I appreciate that Dr. Tianne Foster is bringing so many critical issues to the forefront. It is all too common for staffing issues to be ignored, leaving a heavy burden and expectation to go above and beyond on a daily basis. Working overtime until you are exhausted and skipping meals is considered the norm, not the exception. Reality Check book let me know that I am not alone in this battle against burnout. It is packed full of information and offers valuable strategies and insight.

— Analise Brett, BSPharm, RPh

Dr. Foster, through her book, Reality Check, is addressing one of the largest issues facing healthcare today, the epidemic of clinician burnout. Burnout not only adversely impacts patient care, clinician productivity and quality of care, it dramatically reduces our ability to improve system issues through new processes and innovation adoption. Current attempts to reduce burnout through band-aid solutions, without addressing the deeper issue that result in burnout—a training process that encourages lack of attention to personal emotional needs, a demanding work environment without guardrails to ensure the mental wellness of our healthcare professionals, and an exponential increase in technology that has yet to automate the resultant increased demand in clinician knowledge requirements—cannot adequately resolve the healthcare worker burnout problem. Thank you, Dr. Foster for endeavoring to bring these issues to the forefront.

— Prentice A. Tom, MD
Chief Medical Officer - Kintsugi Health,
Futurist - Vituity Healthcare and Medical Staffing Services.

Equity in medicine or the lack thereof is a topic not frequently discussed. Dr. Foster identifies that biases contribute to burnout. Reality Check does not shy away from discussing the gender bias and racism present in the healthcare industry. It's important to reflect and each do our part to change the organization culture.

— Pringl Miller, MD, FACS
Founder & Executive Director
Physician Just Equity

Medical schools have consistently attracted the most driven, capable, and compassionate individuals from our society, people who genuinely want to make a difference. But as medical students graduate to become doctors, they must contend with a system and culture that expects infallibility, rewards efficiency, and ignores work-life balance. Dr. Foster explores a topic that has always been important yet has remained taboo. Physician burnout is much more prevalent than most would acknowledge, and the consequences to the physician, the physician's family, and patient care are enormous. This is perhaps particularly topical now, as all healthcare workers have had to endure a long pandemic attendant with new risks, more overtime, and attempts to discredit them by those who deny the seriousness of the pandemic. Burnout will threaten the healthcare workforce in general, and it is essential that we understand its causes and devise strategies to address it.

— Oliver F. Bathe, MD, MSc, FRCSC, FACS
Professor of Surgery and Oncology,
University of Calgary, Calgary, Alberta Health Services

REALITY CHECK

RECOGNIZE BURNOUT, PREVENT IT, AND DISCOVER HOW TO LIVE WELL

TIANNE FOSTER, MD

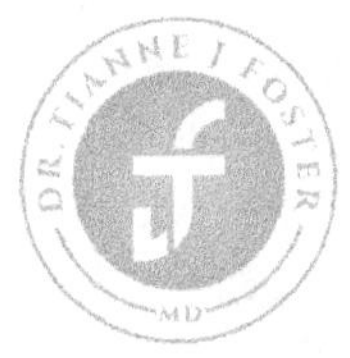

DEDICATION

Dedicated to the selfless professionals, from trainees to seasoned experts, who strive to make a difference, and to those whose lives they touch—may this book offer insights and inspire the collective effort needed for lasting well-being and positive change.

In my experience, it's often the people who are reasonable participants, while the workplace—especially in healthcare—is not. Designing healthcare systems, organizations, and practices that recognize the humanity of those who work within them would be a profound step forward.

— Michael P. Leiter, PhD

Great things are done by a series of small things brought together.

— Vincent van Gogh

TABLE OF CONTENTS

Preface XIII

Introduction 1

Section 1: Too Many Demands and Not Enough Resources 7

    Chapter 1: Relationship Strains 9

    Chapter 2: Work–Life Imbalance 23

    Chapter 3: The Search for Meaning 37

Section 2: Organizational Factors that Contribute to Burnout 43

    Chapter 4: Neglected Needs and Ignored Personal Priorities 45

    Chapter 5: Racial and Ethnic Bias 65

    Chapter 6: Gender Bias 71

    Chapter 7: Unrealistic Expectations 75

    Chapter 8: The Stigma Surrounding Mental Health 83

Section 3: Individual Factors that Contribute to Burnout 91

    Chapter 9: Personality 93

    Chapter 10: Interventions and Coping Methods 111

    Chapter 11: Debt and Financial Burdens 119

Section 4: Consequences of Burnout for the Individual 125

    Chapter 12: Medical Errors 127

    Chapter 13: Exhaustion 135

    Chapter 14: Mental (Un)Wellness 143

Section 5: The Consequences of Burnout for the Patient 163

    Chapter 15: Medical Errors and Disengaged Personnel 165

Section 6: Consequences of Burnout for the Healthcare Organization 171

    Chapter 16: Understanding the Costs of Burnout 173

    Chapter 17: The Cost of Adverse Events 181

Section 7: Addressing Burnout on an Organizational Level 185

Chapter 18: Six Strategies to Address Burnout 187

Conclusion 193

Appendix I: Theoretical Frameworks to Increase Psychological Fortitude and Resilience 197

Remain Resilient in Conflicting Scenarios 199

Remain Resilient in the Presence of Errors 201

Notes 203

References 233

About the Author 273

PREFACE

The discussions in this book reflect studies and statistics available up to 2022—a time when the COVID-19 pandemic was at its peak, reshaping many aspects of our daily lives. That being said, the insights shared here remain timeless and highly relevant.

The strategies and lessons explored are essential for addressing burnout and preventing further distress, especially as we continue to adapt to what is largely considered a post-pandemic world—however long that remains the case. The critical insights within this edition provide actionable steps urgently needed to alleviate burnout.

My hope is that this book serves as a valuable and immediate resource for individuals and organizations committed to preventing burnout and fostering well-being.

INTRODUCTION

"It only gets worse," I was told on two memorable occasions. The first was at my going away celebration a few weeks shy of the start of medical school classes, and the second was in my fourth and final year of medical school during clinical rotations.

I reflect on these two occasions now, realizing not only just how correct those people were, but how blindsided I had been. The major difference in the two encounters was the way each person uttered those words. An ENT (Ear, Nose, and Throat) surgeon who knew the long and trying road that I would have ahead of me, said it the first time with a warm air of endearment. I heard the same words a second time from an emergency physician, likely burned out, who said it in a tone of bitter disgust, demonstrating contempt, cynicism and the lack of gratification or personal accomplishment that he felt in his expansive career. He continued his attempt to convince me and a small group of medical students to switch paths – changing our career trajectories to become nurse practitioners, physician assistants, or anything but physicians. "Get out while you still can!" I remember him saying with an air of gravitas.

We spent an hour of what was to be our weekly didactic teaching session, learning about how "others can make mistakes freely, but regardless of whose mistake it is, at all times the liability will fall on the attending physician".

I remember thinking, *what could have happened to this physician to have drained his joy and corrupted his views so much to place them far from the common desires we usually all start out with as healthcare professionals, that desire to be a helping aide to patients in need'*. Physicians in ancient

Greece swore to uphold the Hippocratic Oath, which has been a doctoral tradition passed down for centuries due to its universal and respected principle. Many medical schools nowadays have adopted a modified version of the Oath that promotes the ethical values of doing no harm and advocating for patients' rights.

Hippocratic Oath: I swear by Apollo the physician, and Asclepius, and Hygieia and Panacea and all the gods and goddesses as my witnesses, that, according to my ability and judgement, I will keep this Oath and this contract:

To hold him who taught me this art equally dear to me as my parents, to be a partner in life with him, and to fulfill his needs when required; to look upon his offspring as equals to my own siblings, and to teach them this art, if they shall wish to learn it, without fee or contract; and that by the set rules, lectures, and every other mode of instruction, I will impart a knowledge of the art to my own sons, and those of my teachers, and to students bound by this contract and having sworn this Oath to the law of medicine, but to no others.

I will use those dietary regimens which will benefit my patients according to my greatest ability and judgement, and I will do no harm or injustice to them.

I will not give a lethal drug to anyone if I am asked, nor will I advise such a plan; and similarly, I will not give a woman a pessary to cause an abortion.

In purity and according to divine law will I carry out my life and my art.

I will not use the knife, even upon those suffering from stones, but I will leave this to those who are trained in this craft.

Into whatever homes I go, I will enter them for the benefit of the sick, avoiding any voluntary act of impropriety or corruption, including the seduction of women or men, whether they are free men or slaves.

Whatever I see or hear in the lives of my patients, whether in connection with my professional practice or not, which ought not to be spoken of outside, I will keep secret, as considering all such things to be private.

So long as I maintain this Oath faithfully and without corruption, may it be granted to me to partake of life fully and the practice of my art, gaining the respect of all men for all time. However, should I transgress this Oath and violate it, may the opposite be my fate. [1]

In the four years following medical school, I began to realize why so many physicians and personnel within the healthcare field lose both their sense of hope in humanity and career satisfaction. In this book, I will present you, the reader, with information that no one taught me anywhere along the trajectory of my medical training. In my experience of medical school, although personal wellness, exercise, and extra-curricular activities were promoted in efforts for us to achieve a good life balance, the most critical purpose for these habits was never discussed.

Indeed, for all the information on how to achieve the ideal balance between work and private life, the overarching question remains: *What exactly are we attempting to ward off?* The dark reality is that the occupational syndrome of burnout is a rampant issue within the healthcare field affecting personnel across virtually every healthcare discipline. And what's more? If nothing is done, it will only get worse!

While searching for a residency training program after medical school, I worked in two different job roles: one was in research as a physician, the second as a healthcare administrative assistant, despite already being trained as a physician. It was in the latter role where I gained invaluable, behind-the-scenes insight into the roles and interplay of physicians, nurses, managers, and administrators. As an administrator, I observed the complex interaction of patients, healthcare professionals, and physicians. Many of my co-workers were unaware of my additional skills and medical background, so my observations provided me with a unique and interesting perspective on the issue of burnout within the healthcare field.

Another event that heightened my curiosity about this widespread issue occurred during a research meeting I took part in during the autumn season, with a surgical trainee. We met at a tall office building adjacent to the main hospital. Working in an office area surrounded by windows, we became distracted, and our conversation soon led to the discussion and admiration of the clear and beautiful view of the city. Although we easily became caught up in admiration of the scenery, I later learned that the aesthetics of this workspace, beautiful as they were, could not deter multiple trainees and doctors from attempting to take their own lives at this location.

I realized early in my career that there was something terribly wrong in the system – a feeling I could not quite shake – thus, I vowed to understand what, why, and how to address it.

Why bring attention to burnout?

Burnout is an occupational syndrome prevalent in society, particularly within *helping* professions such as healthcare. This book aims to provide awareness of what it is and the consequences of it, and to address the risk on the severe end of the spectrum, which is suicide. There will be moments in this book that inspire reactions of pure surprise at the information revealed, much in the same way that I came to these sober realizations. It is an issue experienced in multiple countries, and this book serves to concisely provide information using extensive research that has taken place or been conducted throughout the world. I wholeheartedly believe that people in such roles will be better prepared to overcome the factors leading to burnout if they are made more aware of the issue! Leaders in a position to implement organizational change will be made aware and challenged by the public, professionals, and employees, to urgently enact change.

My heart's desire is that those currently experiencing burnout will discover that there is hope to overcome the challenges that led to its development. If that is you, please know that you are not alone in this situation; myself and many others want to offer our help and understanding.

Together, we can effect change by educating the masses and moving toward the common goal of eradicating burnout by addressing the factors contributing to its development. Make no mistake: burnout can begin during the earliest period of training; this book will prepare students with strategies to handle social conflict and negativity. They will develop awareness of the factors that contribute to burnout, so that they may develop greater resiliency against it. Each lesson stresses the importance of how we evaluate and react to our environment in a situational context; you will learn how to analyze outcomes, whether positive or negative, in the context of individual actions. We should be taught to face reality head on using various strategies to develop ourselves as resilient people.

This book aims to provide a form of a *reality check* regarding the healthcare system and burnout. Although the inner workings of the health system are vast and complex, I will discuss the common factors leading to burnout and suggest how to make adjustments that can, and should be made at the organizational level, the individual healthcare worker level, and consumer level.

Each chapter begins artfully with a quote pulled from real life conversations that provoke discussion on a topic related to burnout. I will address the factors that influence burnout and the consequences of burnout through the discussion of these quotes and the presentation of research findings. I will also explore and elaborate on a strategy to develop positive, constructive thought processes that will help you respond well in the face of tough situations that can lead to burnout.

During these discussions, some details pertaining to identifiable information will be changed to maintain confidentiality.

SECTION 1:
Too Many Demands and Not Enough Resources

Perhaps the most basic cause of burnout is that there are more demands placed upon you as a professional than there are preventative resources within your personal storehouse. A few of the job demands that will be discussed include the administrative burden, excessive workload, moral distress, and inadequate technology/electronic health record (EHR). Let's talk about maintaining meaning in work, having autonomy and job control, quality professional relationships and supportive social interactions.

CHAPTER 1:
RELATIONSHIP STRAINS

"They're the stupidest smart person I know."

Goals: Improve professional relationships and social interaction.

Of course, employees run the risk of burnout across a wide range of demanding occupations, but within healthcare, this issue is pervasive. In a recent consensus study published in the National Academy of Medicine, burnout is defined as an occupational syndrome consisting of a high level of exhaustion (both psychological and emotional), a high level of depersonalization, and a loss of feeling personally accomplished [2]. The prevalence of burnout is noteworthy: between 35 percent to 54 percent of nurses and physicians in the United States have reported symptoms of burnout, and between 45 percent to 60 percent of medical trainees report feeling burned out [3]. Studies have found that the levels of burnout in physicians are higher than that of the general US population [4].

Interestingly, the odds of burnout in a survey of 4000 US physicians, were found to be higher among white physicians compared to physicians of other ethnicities [5]. As one of the first studies to examine burnout among physicians by race and/or ethnicity; their findings of course, have limitations. To start with, the survey could not account for stigma, which is a factor that may lead physicians in minority groups to under-report burnout symptoms. It is also possible that there may be fewer minority physicians expressing burnout due to attrition. Indeed, there are many biases and professional challenges that minority physicians face. There are also many areas where further research is necessary to determine the impact of factors like resilience, life experience, and race or ethnicity on the incidence of burnout.

Speaking of life experiences, a study looking at medical residents in internal medicine found that residents who were considered International Medical Graduates (those who attended a medical school outside the borders of the United States) demonstrated less burnout than their US graduate counterparts [6]. Does the life experience of studying medicine in other countries affect your resilience or vulnerability towards burnout?

The trends within studies have shown that the most vulnerable times for healthcare professionals, seems to be in the beginning of their training or earlier in their careers. In 2017, a survey by the Canadian Medical Association of almost 3,000 resident trainee physicians and physicians, indicated a combined prevalence of burnout of 30 percent [7]. However, there is limited national data regarding burnout in Canadian physicians. Resident trainees

BURNOUT IS DEFINED AS AN OCCUPATIONAL SYNDROME CONSISTING OF A HIGH LEVEL OF EXHAUSTION, DEPERSONALIZATION, AND A LOSS OF FEELING PERSONALLY ACCOMPLISHED.

within the survey demonstrated a higher prevalence of burnout than physicians with a prevalence of 38 percent versus 29 percent respectively. Residents not only indicated higher rates of burnout, they also had increased odds of depression and suicidal ideation [8]. In the Canadian survey, 35 percent of physicians in practice for five years or less had higher reported overall burnout [9]. They had a 45 percent increased risk of experiencing overall burnout than other physicians. What happens when those physicians hit their 6th year of practice? Does their risk of burnout plummet dramatically? No, in fact their risk of burnout only decreased by 13 percent, leaving those physicians with a 32 percent risk in years 6-20 of practice. From year 21- 30 there is a 30 percent risk of burnout and an 18 percent risk for physicians practicing over 30 years [10]. I note these statistics related to length of service in the healthcare field but acknowledge that there is a lack of sufficient research to determine the cause of that trend. The decrease in burnout over time could simply be due to attrition as physicians step out of their medical practice.

Where is burnout most prevalent?

After reviewing research spanning from Scandinavia to Asia, it is clear to me that the issue of burnout among healthcare personnel has become a truly global phenomenon. Merriam-Webster dictionary defines a pandemic as "an outbreak of a disease that occurs over a wide geographic area and affects an exceptionally high proportion of the population." Although burnout is not a disease, we can all agree that it certainly parallels the experience of a pandemic within healthcare personnel.

Obviously, the recent viral pandemic strained workers globally and the healthcare system broadly as demands outpaced resources within the occupation. We know that the causes of burnout are multifactorial. Burnout can be mediated by individual factors and organizational factors in the context of the working environment and culture, each of these components interact as the work system [11]. With that in mind, the next couple of years are critical, and the impact and effects of burnout could become more prevalent if we do not act now to rectify it.

Relationships and Burnout

The relationships we have with the people we work with has a huge bearing on our vulnerability to burnout. A positive relationship with colleagues can mitigate its risk, and a negative one can be a crushing burden to bear daily while increasing the risk of burnout. Multiple studies have demonstrated that difficult professional relationships have been associated with much higher levels of burnout among physicians, nurses, and pharmacists [12]. These challenges, conflicts and stress also exist in interdisciplinary relationships [13]. Studies also show that the perception of conflict also increases when emotionally exhausted, thus demonstrating that deteriorating relationships and burnout are cyclical consequences of each other [14].

> **THE RELATIONSHIPS WE HAVE WITH THE PEOPLE WE WORK WITH HAS A HUGE BEARING ON OUR VULNERABILITY TO BURNOUT.**

Even Unspoken Communication Can Hurt

It is well established that external, non-verbal forms of communication such as body language and demeanor are very impactful. Whether we are conscious of it or not, we can naturally pick up cues about a person's internal affect through their body language. Some studies have estimated that up to 66 percent of communication is non-verbal, while others say that this figure could reach as high as 93 percent [15]. Regardless of which figure is more accurate, *you get the point.* Although someone may not explicitly tell you to your face how incompetent they think you are, their demeanor will surely make it clear. Now, imagine the person who thinks you are incompetent is someone you communicate with every day while you work. With any perceptiveness, you would notice their body language, a condescending tone, or general unfriendliness, all conveyed non-verbally. The fact is that regardless of your education, status, or experience, there will always be someone who thinks poorly of you – this is a form of human nature. There doesn't even have to be a warranted reason *why*, it can be as simple as someone thinking that they have superior insight in comparison to you in one area, resulting in a feeling of being better than you.

The person being discussed in this quote at the beginning of the chapter was a brilliant, top-notch brain surgeon (neurosurgeon), but the topic they were deemed inferior in by their assistant was computers and technology. So that just goes to show, that however brilliant you may be in one area of life, someone more skilled in "Topic 'X'" may use that to their advantage or make themselves feel better by looking down on you.

Let's say your administrator's demeanor changes each time you discuss scheduling, calendars, or emails. By picking up on the non-verbal cues, you may begin to self-reflect on the negativity and conclude that this person has something against you. You may or may not perceive this accurately, although their motives can be unknown.

How would you honestly react to these forms of tense environments? Anyone could experience this at any stage in their careers. Sometimes you may likely be more vulnerable. If you place yourself in the position of the neurosurgeon in that example, would you ignore the person, fire the person and move on, or find something you're better at to hold over that person's head?

I want to give you a strategy to assist in the process of deciding on a course of action that supersedes an instinctive reaction.

A Resiliency framework

A process that I thought-out in advance has helped me to address any difficult social interaction presenting itself, regardless of the way it presents. My hope is that the framework will aid you to devise a personal strategy to find a resolution across a variety of social conflict contexts. I would like you to perceive this framework as a handy toolbox you can access and use to overcome difficult interactions. Indeed, by utilizing these tools, you will develop your resilience. The Merriam-Webster dictionary defines resilience as, 'an ability to recover from or adjust easily to misfortune or change'[16]. Let's discuss how to address social conflicts and interactions using the tools from this framework.

The resiliency framework provides three clarifying questions to ask yourself when assessing how to respond in any scenario:

1. Is this an opinion, or a fact?
2. Does what they think change the reality of how I see myself?
3. Do I have anything to prove?

Fragmenting the framework

It is necessary to break down the framework into fragments so you can better understand it. Question number one is important to address first, because when things are said as an opinion, whether about another person or about a situation, then, by definition, it is not a fact. Reality in and of itself has not changed. The only way that an opinion can change reality is if it is mistakenly categorized as a fact!

For example: You are one of two people looking at a blue shirt and your opinions regarding the color of the shirt may differ, since opinions are formed using evidence that you've built in your own mind about what is in front of you. You state the color of the shirt as blue, but what if we said that the person beside you has some form of color blindness which alters the colors that they can distinguish? That person tells you that they see a green shirt instead of blue. You may or may not know that the person has color blindness, but they tell you that the shirt is green, and without mentioning their medical condition they try to convince you of it.

If you characterize what they've said as their valid opinion which is based on their own evidence, the evidence which you have no access to, then you will continue to make all your conclusions based on your evidence, what your eyes see, and "the shirt is still blue". If, however, in your own mind you characterize that what they said about the color of the shirt being green is a fact regardless of understanding the evidence, then you will likely begin to question what you are seeing with your own eyes. You'll question your own reality, and over time you might assume that the blue color you saw was wrong. The inability to accurately distinguish opinion from fact, could lead to decreased personal autonomy.

Applying the Resiliency framework

Now, let's apply that to a workplace context of when someone is speaking about your work ethic, knowledge, personality, or skill, and let's review the scenario between the neurosurgeon and administrator. Putting yourself in the shoes of the neurosurgeon, you could answer the first question about whether the statement is a fact or an opinion one of two ways. Perhaps the administrator provided convincing evidence of your poor computer literacy through a few examples, or you are already aware of your deficiencies. In such cases, you could conclude that yes, it is a *fact* that you are bad at navigating computer technology.

Regardless, answering the first question that you are dealing with a "fact" in and of itself does not yet determine the best response. So, let's answer the next question in our framework: "Does what they think change the reality of how I see myself?" Remember, our personal reality refers to the way that we see ourselves. My reality or opinion of myself can become affected by my priorities.

Back to the neurosurgeon scenario, you can now ask yourself whether it is your priority to become better at computer technology. If yes, then the framework evokes a natural response to dedicate more time to studying computers. If that's not your priority, especially if it is not within your scope of interests or a significantly useful skill to you, then your conclusion might be to increase your surgical knowledge and improve patient care.

The next question in the framework helps determine our action: "Do I have anything to prove?" By answering, you can easily determine if a reply or any further thought on the subject is warranted. Do you want to prove to the antagonist in this scenario that you are in fact great at computers? Is it important to set the person straight or to clarify to them that you are working hard towards that particular priority? If your answer here is "No" then the solution is to brush the tense interaction aside. Brushing the conflict aside includes refraining from reacting to that person's comments or condescending behavior.

Many of us don't like to let anyone "get away with" condescending comments about our abilities or capabilities. However, greater conflict usually arises when we give precedence and rebuttal to trivial matters.

Why is this important? As seen in the research, those with even a perception of a negative relationship in the workplace, regardless of whether or not that perception was accurate, demonstrated increased levels of burnout [17]. These findings applied to nurses and all other members of the healthcare team, where relationships and communication with other staff members have shown critical importance; negative relationships correlate with increased levels of burnout [18].

The best, high-quality relationships in the workplace integrate shared goals, shared knowledge, and mutual respect. This necessarily includes frequent and accurate communication that aims to solve problems in a timely manner. Termed as Relational Coordination, the image below shows these components, and the interaction that increases performance, quality and safety [19].

I encourage you to be truly intentional in adopting this thought process framework. Use it with and for purpose. It will decrease negative perceptions and therefore serve to decrease your risks of burnout.

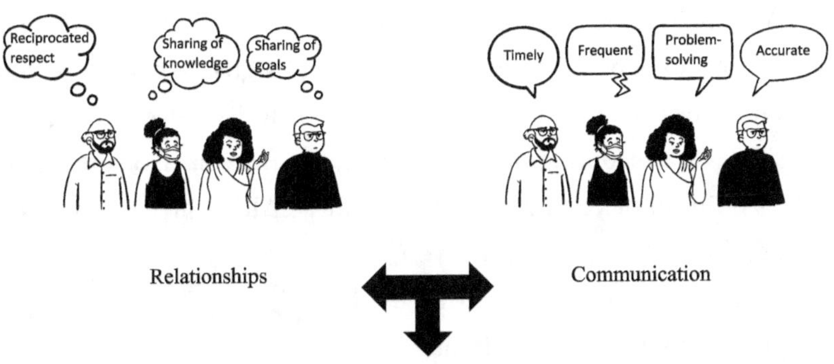

Increased performance, quality, and safety

A Trivial Conflict

I came across the story of two people in conflict who had once been very good friends; when they paused to reflect and discuss what led to the tension, they realized it was the result of something trivial. Sometimes disagreements are provoked, not so much about differing viewpoints, but by one person's manner of reactivity that went against how the other person expected to be treated. In summary, as you answer each of the questions, if something does not change your personal reality, and does not require proving a particular point, then read carefully: it does not warrant a response, *period.*

What others think of you is none of your business

There are two relevant quotes from motivational speakers that come to mind. The first is "What others think of you is none of your business", meaning that until someone verbalizes what they're thinking, you should not make any assumptions or be concerned over it. We can't judge or make assumptions based solely on non-verbal signs. When we're concerned, it is always better to ask the person to clarify before jumping to conclusions. The second quote comes from Les Brown, "Don't let someone else's opinion of you become your reality". Although someone may verbalize their thoughts about you, you are under no obligation to take their opinions to heart and in doing so change your opinion of yourself. These principles are so important when faced with negativity and conflict – even beyond the confines of the clinic.

> **WHAT OTHERS THINK OF YOU IS NONE OF YOUR BUSINESS.**

Self-Reflection in the Context of Relationships

One self-care author described psychological health as self-awareness and self-knowledge, but personally speaking, I believe that psychological health represents much more than that. For instance, it must also include the awareness of yourself in relation to others, and an awareness and knowledge of how others are relating to you. Simply put, we should know psychologically how we are affected by others and our effect on others too. Do you tend to react to others quickly and defensively, passively, or considerately? When you speak to others are you brash, condescending, empathetic, or personable? This is important to be aware of, because how reactive you are will affect not only yourself, but those around you too. Sometimes, we escalate conflict unknowingly because of the body language and tone we adopt due to strong emotions. When we pause, for even a short time and mentally work through the framework, strong emotions dissipate and we can develop a constructive response, with the appropriate tone and physical demeanor.

At the end of the day, we should treat others the way we would want to be treated.

Know thyself

If you don't already, it is necessary to have firm convictions of your identity and self-worth. Cultivating that confidence takes time and honest reflection – with which you must challenge your self-critical or negative thinking in order to renew the mind with new habits of thinking that develop the positive framework we all need.

Using the framework will help you accept constructive criticisms, as well as make you more capable of accepting factual critiques you can take to heart and improve upon. It is a useful life habit, to pause for self-reflection before social conflicts develop or fester. Pausing helps us to create space between incidents and our reactions to them – and this space can be useful for thinking before we act, as well as applying the critical resiliency framework as mentioned earlier. Collect facts and ask yourself questions such as: *How do I tend to treat others, what is my work ethic, do I give tasks my full effort, do I conduct myself ethically, and do I portray a positive demeanor?* Reflecting on your true identity, not basing your identity on the opinions of others, will help establish the confidence you need before going into difficult social interactions. For example, if people are commenting on your work ethic, you should have already developed confidence based on your track record and values you embrace during times of reflection. You should know how hard you work and use that as a benchmark to distinguish between opinions versus facts.

Consistent self-reflection and use of the framework will prepare you to distinguish between fact and opinion. If people say things that contradict your values and conclusions, you may be prompted to ask them for examples or evidence that may reveal any blind spots you've possibly overlooked.

Remember to utilize the framework and do not let someone else's opinion of you determine your reality.

Key Chapter Points

- A positive relationship can mitigate burnout, or a negative relationship can become a burnout risk.
- The most impactful forms of communication are often given by external cues, which are the non-verbal forms of communication such as body language and demeanor.

- Utilize the resiliency framework

  - Three questions to ask when assessing how to respond in a situation are:

    - Is this an opinion or fact?
    - Does what they think change the reality of how I see myself?
    - Do I have anything to prove?

- Don't let a trivial conflict ruin a relationship.
- What others think of you is none of your business!
- Know thyself

  - Don't let someone else's opinion of you become your reality!

- Be prepared and confident by practicing self-reflection in advance of any conflicts.

CHAPTER 2:
WORK–LIFE IMBALANCE

"Why can't I just pay to have this done faster?
I can do that at the passport office."

---

*Goals: **Decrease administrative burden and respect clinician time and autonomy.***

A study reviewing a subgroup of American physicians in the specialty of outpatient family medicine, found that they spent 4.5 hours on average during clinic on the Electronic Health Record (EHR) and another 1.4 hours after their final patient completing chart review, documentation, and managing messages within the EHR. This length of time equates to almost half of their day; the average day within the study was 11.4 hours [20]. Additionally, they spent an hour of their time on the EHR on weekends. This study did not consider physicians who also carried out work with inpatients at the hospital.

There are pros and cons with the addition of the electronic health record (EHR). While it is intended to share information from patient care across locations and disciplines in a convenient way, there must be more focus shifted to the patient-physician interaction, which represents the ultimate purpose of patient care. Originally, EHRs were set up as a tool for billing, coding, and protection from litigation. Its pros include improved easy review of the patient history, and a superior medication prescription system that has alerts built in to decrease medication errors [21].

Of course, improvements in the integration of healthcare and technology are necessary, but the EHR system has some serious issues. From its poor interface which does not match clinical workflow limits, and the lack of quality individualized care, to the extensive documentation – the system requires and consumes so much of the time of highly skilled personnel [22].

Safety alerts have their own pros and cons, as multiple alerts and reminders can be generated for patients with many chronic conditions. "Alert fatigue" can lead to missed important information, workflow interruptions, and unhealthy distractions for personnel [23]. Extensive documentation throughout the chart leads to information overload [24]. Increased risk of burnout is therefore a natural consequence of these problems when combined with low physician satisfaction [25]. Better EHR technology is desperately needed, and clinicians should be involved in these developments, if not the driving force leading the endeavor. Technologies that could provide accurate, predictive analytics, allow for more individualized patient care, and improved outcomes that would greatly reduce burnout.

The Continuing Education Burden

Not only do the ongoing requirements within the EHR encroach on clinician time outside of working hours, but many clinicians must also complete mandatory yearly education modules required by regulators or take ongoing continuing medical education (CME) to maintain certifications. Most organizations provide neither time off to help facilitate this, nor compensation to salaried healthcare professionals for these requirements.

This means that physicians that teach and train our future healthcare workers must often meet the requirements for scholarly activity on per-

sonal time. Academic medical centers set criteria for required educational responsibilities and publications while allocating little or no time for
these endeavors. In fact, for these physicians, performance requirements
for clinical care have remained the same or increased.

All of these pressures on the balance between work and personal life lead
to increased burnout among clinicians, not only due to the added workload and burdens but also due to moral distress. A serious moral disconnect can happen when clinicians have little or no autonomy concerning
tasks that they deem are not critical to patient care. I've already alluded
to excessive documentation being among these tasks [26]. Work that en-
croaches into personal time also gives the employing organization a false
sense of increased productivity, when really, the organization's additional
measures are being met at the cost of stolen time and pay from clinicians,
without assessing the impact on patient care and clinician well-being.

Restricting Hours

In 2003, the USA's Accreditation Council for Graduate Medical Education (ACGME) implemented work hour adjustments to not only address
training physician fatigue, but to also improve patient safety [27]. Trainees were restricted to 80-hour work weeks and limited to 30 hours for
continuous shifts. What's been the impact on educational satisfaction or
fatigue? [28]. In some studies the prevalence of burnout decreased, showing
less emotional exhaustion on the Maslach Burnout Inventory [29]. Some
have thought that the hours restrictions might limit the time trainees
and attending physicians have to spend on teaching opportunities [30]. It's
possible that work which would have been done by trainees prior to the
restriction, would be passed on to attending physicians, thus increasing
their workload. Or worse, it's possible perhaps that the workload itself

would not decrease at all, so the same amount of work would be expected to be completed within an even shorter amount of time.

On clinical rotations as a medical student, I recall moments when the attending physician would take time to teach during patient interactions and the resident physicians would leave to complete their charting or orders for their patients. Observational studies have shown that since the implementation of the work hours restrictions, interns spent less time in direct care of patients and less time sleeping [31]. The number of administrative tasks that are required to be completed for each patient in conjunction with work hour restrictions, takes away from the patient interaction and thus learning opportunities. The observational study from 2013 found that a sample of intern residents were seen to spend eight minutes or less with each patient. Twelve percent of their time was in direct patient contact, and 64 percent of their time involved completing orders, communicating with other staff, and writing notes [32]. Fifteen percent of their time was used for education, and 9 percent for activities such as eating, sleeping, walking, and recreation. Forty percent of their time was spent in front of a computer screen, typically reviewing patient charts. Let's be honest here, these are alarming statistics! Less patient interaction may not be due to work hour restrictions, but rather a combination of factors, including the extensive time required for administrative tasks.

> **SINCE THE IMPLEMENTATION OF THE WORK HOURS RESTRICTIONS, INTERNS SPENT LESS TIME IN DIRECT CARE OF PATIENTS AND LESS TIME SLEEPING.**

Could compassion be the clear fix?

One author of a book addressing improving well-being for health professionals described what they thought was a simple solution to combat the inherent difficulties resulting in burnout. Their solution was this: to be more compassionate. The healthcare profession was described as a field of compassion, and surely with more compassion, it would benefit everyone – right?

You might be inclined to agree, but perhaps the bigger question is, *compassion towards who?* Obviously, healthcare professionals must exercise their compassion towards suffering patients and families. But who shows compassion towards them?

 Perhaps many of the issues contributing to burnout would disappear if, over time, everyone in the system including the organizational administration exercised compassion and more specifically, empathy. Empathy is defined as "the action of understanding, being aware of, being sensitive to, and vicariously experiencing the feelings, thoughts, and experience of another of either the past or present without having the feelings, thoughts, and experience fully communicated in an objectively explicit manner" [33]. I'll paraphrase that! Empathy is to place yourself in someone else's shoes in order to understand what they are experiencing.

Affording empathy to another is a complex process involving many factors, however – and can actually result in more personal distress [34]. To empathize and express caring concern with less personal distress, the key is imagining the other person's feelings in their situation rather than imagining yourself in the situation. Compassion is defined as "sympathetic consciousness of others' distress together with a desire to alleviate it" [35], also synonymous with words such as pity, and sympathy.

I agree with the author that it would be helpful if organizations stepped back to consider how they can keep compassionate patient care as their primary goal. Organizations and their staff must be intentional and united in pursuing this as a common goal to successfully communicate compassion toward patients.

After all, when staff disconnect over time from their primary sense of compassion a shift to cynicism and depersonalization from burnout can set in. Every healthcare organization wants its staff to successfully pursue that mutual and all-important primary goal, compassionate patient care. Thus, it is imperative that staff are treated and nurtured in a way that promotes worker engagement instead of promoting over-working and burnout.

When it comes to the EHR and those excessive administrative burdens discussed earlier, organizations themselves should become empathetic towards their staff needs and strive to understand how poor technologies and administrative burdens contribute to burnout and ultimately sabotage the common goal of compassionate patient care. Technology developers should also take an empathetic note to ensure that their technological advancements are developed with compassionate care programmed into their coding, to improve patient outcomes, communication, and efficiency.

Act Without Expectation

Of course, people who enter the healthcare profession should be compassionate; educators should help them to both develop and display empathy. These skills should be nurtured and perfected in practice. However, when considering burnout, the "compassion solution" may be too simplistic. The fact is that in the general population, there will of course be some people who are not empathetic and may not even be considerate! From a young age, human beings are self-focused and primarily concerned with self-preservation, and they must be taught to consider others. Don't oversimplify or naively assume that others will return your display of compassion. Such expectations lead to inevitable disappointments. You cannot base your compassionate actions and response to others on an unhealthy expectation of receiving the same in return. Practicing compassion and acts of kindness without strings of expectation has been shown to aid in increasing our overall level of happiness [36]. While displaying acts of kindness towards others, you can't assume that other people are at the same emotional level or ability to demonstrate compassion or empathy.

In summary, remaining empathetic and compassionate to others without expecting reciprocation is not easy. Working with multiple patients of varying personalities and complaints can challenge composure as well as compassion. Staff members can become emotionally exhausted, eroding their ability to act compassionately, display sympathy or respect, becoming detached and possibly calloused [37].

> **YOU CANNOT BASE YOUR COMPASSIONATE ACTIONS AND RESPONSE TO OTHERS ON AN UNHEALTHY EXPECTATION OF RECEIVING THE SAME IN RETURN.**

People in positions in human services, whether healthcare, social services, law enforcement and so on, often face and experience strong emotions. Embarrassment, fear, and frustration can be felt by both the client and professionals. Clients or patients present problems to be solved, focusing on the negative aspects of their lives and situations. The discussion, by design, rarely mentions the positive aspects of those patients' lives. Healthcare professionals can then unconsciously view those patients in a negative light. It is possible to either over-identify with them and sympathize or dissociate and alienate the patient or client. Complex conditions or adverse personalities can also come into play, adding to the strong emotions for the professional.

Over time, if you don't develop an ability to cope with such strong emotions, particularly if you don't see tangible gratification in your career, you may become emotionally exhausted [38]. Burnout in relation to empathy may directly correlate with your ability to shift your focus away from the self to others when those negative emotions arise as you witness patients in distress [39]. Empathy is extremely complex, but it need not result in personal distress.

Some in human service professions regulate their emotions through a form of detached concern [40], whereby they attempt to distance themselves from their emotions while also trying to remain concerned for the patient or client [41]. This particular practice is painted by others as a form of emotional regulation: controlling emotions to protect against a more stressful and intense emotional crisis [42]. Halpern describes detached concern as very different than empathy [43]. However, Lampert and Glaser describe the *concern* component of detached concern as empathic concern, demonstrating compassion and acting to decrease another's suffering [44].

Studies have shown that low detachment and low concern coincide with the highest levels of burnout [45]. Along the same line, the highest emotional exhaustion was apparent when the level of concern was high, with low detachment. High depersonalization was seen when detachment was higher than levels of concern. I found a fascinating study of 7,584 practicing physicians in Latin America with similar findings [46]. Physicians with alexithymia – which is an unawareness and inability to describe their own emotions – exhibited a correlation with higher personal distress and higher rates of burnout along with secondary traumatic stress. They also had significantly lower levels of empathetic concern. This research into the relationship between empathy and burnout is ongoing. Some have seen a negative correlation, meaning that when one was high the other was low [47], but further research is needed into their relationship, connection, and the factors that can affect change.

Is healthcare just a complex passport office?

Whether it is intentional or not, people have the tendency to mentally group their experiences together and derive their expectations, conclusions, or opinions from their previous experiences. When someone expects to receive service, they may group all service providing industries together. This is certainly the case within the healthcare services too.

In one scenario, an individual came to the physician's office and expected the same form of service as they would at their passport office. Someone might argue that there are similarities, such as conforming to established standards and best practices of customer service – but there are obvious differences which will become apparent. A patient's family member approached a clinic receptionist, demanding that a physician letter and insurance paperwork completed by the following day. Physicians receive multiple documents and notes to accurately complete daily (not including the EHR tasks), none of which can be delegated to a hired staff member without the appropriate credentials. Such a demand on a healthcare professional, lacks not only empathy but also understanding. *This is not the passport office.*

STUDIES HAVE SHOWN THAT LOW DETACHMENT AND LOW CONCERN COINCIDE WITH THE HIGHEST LEVELS OF BURNOUT.

This lack of understanding has even infiltrated the language we use to describe physicians, nurses, and clinicians – grouped together in one category as "healthcare providers". The notion of a "healthcare provider" is one which implies that these professionals exist simply to "provide" whatever "health care" is needed by the customer, in this case the patient. Whether the "need" is for a prescription or otherwise, the term "provider" devalues the insight, knowledge, and judgment obtained over the extensive years of training as a healthcare professional. Those are the basis for recommending the best courses of action. To reduce such a diverse range of roles, each with their own distinct training, to the blanket term of "healthcare provider" can certainly blur the lines of their varied scope of practice.

In an article written in Forbes by Bruce Y. Lee, he mentioned an unfortunate comparison a healthcare consulting firm partner made between a hospital and a fast-food restaurant [48]. The notion that patients can pull up to a clinic or hospital with the same mind-set as if they are pulling up to a fast-food drive-thru is simply unnerving. The idea propagates that healthcare professionals are meant to simply provide patients with whatever their requests or orders may be, which is transforming our healthcare system into a factory producing burnout victims.

Sure, clinicians do provide many things for their patients – in terms of advice, insight, and expert knowledge; however, they are much more than providers. They are also advocates and confidants that patients often value and respect.

This level of respect and value begin to breakdown when this relationship is generalized into one of a "provider and client/patient" (or worse: 'customer,') like that of a customer and server in a McDonald's chain restaurant. The only similarity may be that demands often run high in both environments, but the danger in this 'provider' mindset is the old saying or the notion that "the customer is always correct". The idea is that whatever the customer wants is in their best interest. That might be true in a restaurant, but not necessarily in healthcare. Indeed, patients in the healthcare system are not "customers" in the traditional sense.

Each treatment, test, and option have pros and cons which need to be weighed with many physiological implications in mind. A simple blood test is not so simple when you consider the implications of what a result could indicate! Why is a blood test warranted? Is it sensitive or specific enough to test for the condition of interest? Would the results imply steps to manage the issue revealed? Among all these considerations are the very important factors of the cost for each investigation, action, or treatment.

Do you see how dangerous the *fast-food mentality* within healthcare can be?

Physicians are supposed to offer patients their expert opinion and inform them of the various options for care and investigation, and in doing so, allow their patients to make an informed decision. However, the fast-food restaurant mentality is propagated through healthcare organizations that have implemented time constraints and increased patient load. Physicians are expected to make a quick assessment, diagnose, and treat and advise within a narrowed timeframe. Empathetic and informed discussion is critical to allow shared decision making in this clinician-patient relationship. It may be critical and expected, yet it's placed to the backburner with all of these restrictive time constraints.

Clinicians working under these time pressures, requirements, and performance measures are soon forced to adapt to the 'fast-food' type of healthcare, adding to the systemic breakdown. No wonder there is such moral distress for these clinicians who are forced to adjust to requirements which leads to less and less face time with patients, a critical component of their medical training and one of the deepest, heartfelt desires that motivated them to healthcare in the first place.

In some countries, the ever increasing direct-to-consumer advertisements by large pharmaceutical companies only adds to the minimization of the clinician role. Pharmaceuticals spend billions of dollars advertising medications which have minimal use within the broader population. In the 'fast-food healthcare system,' clinicians sometimes begin to practice defensive medicine out of fear of litigation or complaints.

Within this growing mentality of 'fast-food' healthcare, there also is the notion that healthcare personnel are interchangeable. As in the fast-food industry, restaurant servers are interchangeable, so too in organizations says this mentality. This minimizes the significant training, skill, and role differences of healthcare personnel. A nurse will not provide the same insight as a physician and vice versa. These different healthcare personnel soon become grouped into one term – *healthcare provider* – but they each have a different skillset.

> **THE FAST-FOOD RESTAURANT MENTALITY IS PROPAGATED THROUGH HEALTHCARE ORGANIZATIONS THAT HAVE IMPLEMENTED TIME CONSTRAINTS AND INCREASED PATIENT LOAD.**

Let's maintain these distinctions instead of allowing ambiguous terms like 'provider' to decrease role definitions and clarity that are important for patients, organizations, and the general public to understand.

The term of Advanced Practice Provider is an ambiguous example, also called Advanced Clinical Practitioner in the UK. This term could refer to a nurse practitioner, physician assistant, pharmacist, or therapist to name a few [49]. Each of these roles has complex scopes of practice that are in fact very different. Considering the push to increase the number of 'advanced practice providers' within the healthcare system – I must ask, *what improvements to the system is in mind?*

Unfortunately, administrative demands don't change based on the scope of a professional's particular practice. Anyone in patient care is still expected to complete extensive insurance and authorization forms, detracting from the time important to patient care. The best use of clinician time is not completing hours of paperwork; however, in the fast-food mentality the first adjustments made involve taking physicians away from patient care; physicians are replaced completely with one or multiple 'advanced practice practitioners.' Instead of considering how to minimize menial tasks in order to improve patient care, organizations aim to cut costs instead of increase efficiency.

Administrative burdens clearly take away from the time for quality patient care and leads to greater amounts of burnout. Replacements with advanced practitioners will not resolve this issue. It would be best to have a compassionate approach that aligns with logic: preventing burnout and improving healthcare management cuts costs and decreases staff turnover.

In summary, empathy could go a long way to help halt the deterioration of the healthcare system and the growing problem of burnout. Empathy would enable administrators and organizations to develop a deep understanding of the burnout issue from the healthcare professional perspective. This improved understanding would logically show that healthcare professionals too, as extensive as their training is, have basic human needs, and that the host of administrative assignments they are subjected to are not essential to their most critical role.

Key Chapter Points

- Remain empathetic and compassionate towards others without expecting reciprocation.
- Clinicians should have autonomy and respected personal time outside of work hours.
- Technological advancements should improve compassionate care, communication, and efficiency.
- The 'fast-food' mentality and ambiguous terminology such as 'healthcare provider' should be avoided.

CHAPTER 3:
THE SEARCH FOR MEANING

"Being in the operating room is the only place I can catch a break."

Goals: Activate resources, find meaning in work, improve job control, and balance the workload.

To be inspired, engaged, and most effective at work, people must believe that the work that they are doing has inherent meaning. Surveys indicate that having meaning in work or a 'sense of calling' is associated with less burnout and more engagement [50]. By 'engagement', I'm referring to precisely the opposite of burnout – and by 'meaning', we're talking about a sense of accomplishment and importance that brings joy and feelings of success and fulfillment from work. Unfortunately, surveys of healthcare staff about whether they have joy or meaning in their work reveal dismal results, this, in a profession in which no matter the discipline (medicine, nursing, or pharmacy), people placed a high value on meaning and purpose, which would lower the rates of burnout [51].

The Maslach Burnout Inventory measure (MBI) indicated that 71 percent of emergency medicine physicians in Israel were burned out. Worries and lack of meaning in their roles contributed to that burnout [52]. The worries expressed fell across 3 chief areas:

HAVING MEANING IN WORK OR A 'SENSE OF CALLING' IS ASSOCIATED WITH LESS BURNOUT AND MORE ENGAGEMENT.

stress from strained relationships with other staff or unprofessional staff, worries about negative (abusive or impolite) interactions from patients and families, and stress related to the dysfunctional management of the healthcare system they worked in. In contrast, emergency physicians found meaning from interesting cases and diversity of their specialty, and positive relationships with other team members, patients and their families. It was genuine excitement and satisfaction that those physicians reported when they knew they had contributed to society, made a correct diagnosis, and impacted or saved lives – their antidote to burnout.

Studies of 'Meaning' in US physicians

Sixty-five percent of Internal Medicine physicians in the US indicated that patient care was the aspect of work that added the most meaning for them, while others indicated research (19 percent), education (9 percent), and administration (3 percent) as the most meaningful [53]. Interestingly, physicians who spent less than one day per week, (~20 percent) of their time in the area they found most meaningful, experienced greater burnout (53.8 percent vs. 29.9 percent).

As for gender and age differences, women (43 percent vs. 31 percent) and physicians less than 55 years old (42.3 percent vs. 20.7 percent) had higher burnout rates, this was independent from the time spent in their area of meaning. Within the group surveyed, internal medicine subspecialists were likely to spend at minimum 20 percent of their time on the activity of most interest as opposed to general internists [54]. Those generalists within the group were more likely to experience burnout (42.3 percent vs. 20.7 percent). Not surprisingly, those who were experiencing burnout were more likely to express their intention to leave their position or make a cut back to only part-time hours.

The correlation between levels of burnout and lack of work meaning are very clear.

Engagement in the United Kingdom

In the UK, the National Health Service (NHS) Employers organization works with the NHS to maintain an engaged and sustainable workforce [55]. Three different offices within the NHS Employers organization participate in this effort: the National Engagement Service, the office of Development and Employment, and Employment Relations and Reward.

The National Engagement Service aims to improve effective organization and patient care quality [56]. In 2018, the Institute for Employment Studies (IES), commissioned by NHS Employers, evaluated the link between the engagement of staff and positive patient experience in North East England [57]. They concluded that the two are closely tied; staff experience deeply affects patient experience. The organization recognized that staff members, particularly those who do not directly work in patient care, need to be encouraged that their work matters to the overall patient experience. They acted on those findings to direct staff focus to patient care, taking measures such as providing ample positive and negative feedback from patients in a timely manner, and upholding the primary value of patients first. Realizing that staff shortages put pressure on frontline workers and affects patients, HR departments worked hard to recruit staff faster, which not only alleviated some staffing pressures, but also reduced spending from the agency [58].

Areas of Meaning

The surgeon who said "Being in the operating room is the only place I can catch a break" revealed where he found the most meaning and psychological freedom. He went even further and expressed that if he was unable to have adequate time in the operating room, then his medical career was not worthwhile. It was those moments in the operating room that he found his niche, experienced fulfillment and in some respects experienced 'self-actualization,' the term Maslow coined in his hierarchy, to be discussed in Section 2 Chapter 1.

Because the healthcare field is so focused on others, it is especially important to pause and reflect regularly on what aspects of your work are most fulfilling and provide you with the most energy and meaning. A sense of meaning in the healthcare profession is a powerful preventative against burnout. Meaning can be felt inwardly as a strong sense of reward, in addition to job control, connection with others, and respect. The external reward brought by praise and positive feedback on the job is also a viable deterrent against burnout [59].

And let's not forget the impact that financial compensation makes to alleviate burnout statistics. Debt and the worry about future compensation are potential grave contributors to the increased risk for burnout [60]. A study of 900 physicians, and a study of 26,000 nurses, both showed that income did not account for differences in levels of staff burnout [61]. Other studies found a connection between compensation with increased rates of burnout [62]. A study of 602 Canadian nurses and 974 clinical pharmacists found that if they perceived an unfair level of rewards and appreciation compared to their work effort, burnout increased [63].

These indicate at least a psychological component to forms of monetary compensation that can impact burnout. Workers need to feel appreciated; and when in debt, the worry about future compensation can impact their current mental wellbeing. McHugh and colleagues found, however, that for nurses in a poor work and staffing environment, higher wages was not the primary factor driving their levels of burnout, although it did impact job satisfaction and intents to leave [64].

Key Chapter Points

- Engagement is considered an opposite entity to burnout, and can be optimized through meaning; developing a sense of accomplishment and importance within a person's work tasks.
- Burnout may be related to debt worry, and perceived imbalance between effort, contributions and appreciation or fair compensation.

SECTION 2:
Organizational Factors that Contribute to Burnout

It is ironic that within healthcare, the very factors that contribute to burnout are inadvertently promoted within the organizational culture. Indeed, poor staff coverage, extreme patient load or clinic demands, and implicit/explicit biases all promote imbalanced and unhealthy work lifestyle behaviors. Violence is an all-too-common occurrence. Clinician wellness can be at odds with what is considered *good* employee behavior. If within an organizational culture, a physician who takes breaks, vacations, or seeks support from others whether professional or personal, is seen as rare and thus unnatural, that physician may soon be labeled as 'bad', unprofessional, or lacking in work ethic. These ideas only serve to enable burnout and need to be challenged!

CHAPTER 4:
NEGLECTED NEEDS AND IGNORED PERSONAL PRIORITIES

"He's a staff doctor now, right? He can suck
it up; he's expected to pick up the slack."

Goals: Respect and ensure basic human rights are upheld.

Depending on the country, physicians in their first few years of practice report a higher incidence of burnout compared to their more senior counterparts. This may seem surprising – after all, a narrow understanding of burnout may imply that you've been working a long time and become burned out from it. Well, as it turns out, the answer isn't that simple.

In Canada, burnout rates varied little with years of experience in practice, between 30 to 35 percent, those in practice for fewer years having a slightly higher percentage with burnout [65]. In the USA, physicians between 40 to 54 years old reported higher burnout levels than their counterparts who were either younger or older [66]. This result may be due to time juggling many roles caring for children, aging parents, and planning their own retirements. In the United Kingdom, statistics on burnout levels remained consistently around 40 percent until dropping off after the mid-fifties [67].

Where the early stages of a physician's career can be vulnerable to a high risk for burnout, it could be due to the imbalance between demands and resources, likely to be higher at the start of a career.

I overheard "He's a staff doctor now, right? He can suck it up; he's expected to pick up the slack," made as a passing comment by an administrator organizing a new staff physician's clinic. That statement reflects the often unspoken and very unreasonable demands placed upon new physician hires and other healthcare trainees. There is great pressure on new staff members to yield to these expectations as 'part of the new role,' not to mention fearing repercussion from colleagues or superiors for expressing any apprehension.

That administrator's misconception—that it is okay to overwork, over-schedule, and overlook the value of new hires—is all too common, and not exclusive to the healthcare field. When anyone attains success beyond what is considered average achievement, society tends to project upon that person superhuman levels of responsibility and ability. This is especially true among highly esteemed professions like physicians, lawyers, professional athletes, business executives and prosperous entrepreneurs. People in such roles are often held to very high standards which is understandable and natural – after all, the word professional ascribes a certain level of competence and integrity – but soon the superhuman expectations diminish their basic human needs and exaggerate their basic human capacities. When certain people are elevated to a *superhuman* category, it's easier, then, to justify neglecting them.

Superheroes Never Need Breaks

You've never watched a movie in which Superman, Wonder Woman, or Thor, took a bathroom break or a mid-day lunch break to eat and hydrate, while battling to save the world. These heroes are never exhausted, physically or emotionally; they handle whatever is thrown their way – and when they appear to be beaten up and you think they might be down and out – they summon the strength to bounce right back and save the day.

Those who were on the frontlines working against the effects of COVID-19 serve as a profound and relevant example of a group publicly deemed as *superhuman*. Healthcare workers were called superheroes long before this global crisis, which can predispose them to being over-worked through difficult conditions like the Coronavirus pandemic. While it is true that nobody possesses superhuman abilities, due to the unde-niable hard-work, ethics and sacrifices of healthcare personnel, society may see the intense efforts, particularly giv-en in a crisis, and assume that this same intensity will simply be the new normal.

YOU'VE NEVER WATCHED A MOVIE IN WHICH SUPERMAN, WONDER WOMAN, OR THOR, TOOK A BATHROOM BREAK OR A MID-DAY LUNCH BREAK TO EAT AND HYDRATE, WHILE BATTLING TO SAVE THE WORLD.

Irrespective of whether the hard-work ethic or the *superhuman label* be-comes a healthcare worker's normal lifestyle, the fact is that healthcare staff still have basic human needs. To delve deeper into the discussion of human needs and how they manifest in our private life and our occupa-tions, it is necessary to introduce *Maslow's hierarchy of needs*.

Abraham Maslow was an American psychologist who identified a ba-sic hierarchy of human needs in 1943 [68]. He depicted this hierarchy in pyramid form, comprised of five distinct levels of 'needs,' with the most fundamental needs delineated at its base and 'self-actualization' as the ultimate goal atop the apex. The needs sandwiched in between the base of physiological needs and the apex of self-actualization are safety, be-longingness, and esteem.

We could continue the ongoing debate about whether these levels represent steppingstones – whereby people move from one level to the next in a unilateral direction – or if a person can experience self-actualization as more of a fluid process moving back and forth on the pyramid.

The physiological needs are what Maslow termed 'deficiency needs,' meaning that if these are not met, an individual will experience inner conflict, becoming anxious, tense, and unable to progress in life or reach their full potential. These fundamental and universal physiological needs include food, shelter, clothing, and homeostasis (an inner balance or stability).

Maslow proposed that when people are fulfilled in one level, they are then motivated to level up and focus on the next levels in succession. With this context in mind, the next level on the pyramid after the physiological base is that of safety, which includes personal security, emotional and financial stability, health, and well-being. Above that is love and belonging, which represents the human need for interpersonal relationships such as friendships that foster intimacy, trust, and affiliation with a group. Maslow positioned esteem needs at the fourth level, encompassing qualities like dignity, achievement, independence, and the esteem derived from others – including respect, reputation, appreciation, and prestige. He placed self-actualization at the top of the hierarchy, describing this as the need for a high level of personal fulfillment and satisfaction in what they are best suited for.

Maslow acknowledged that the order shown in the pyramid might be flexible and based on one's unique environment and individual differences. Some proponents of this hierarchy model have, over the years, proposed adding more levels to the pyramid – to include factors like cognitive needs, aesthetic needs, and transcendence at the top of the hierarchy. While there are critics of the hierarchy created by Maslow, we can generally accept that these needs do widely correlate with the human condition across every culture. It is universally acknowledged that unmet needs, can produce inner conflict.

The point of this discussion with respect to healthcare superhumans is that once society determines that you have achieved success, and subconsciously conclude that you have reached the pinnacle of self-actualization – they're likely to forget or disregard the ongoing more fundamental needs you require on a daily basis.

Developmental Models of Burnout

Maslow's hierarchy has simply been presented here to add clarity on how burnout might occur in the world of healthcare, although it doesn't portray that directly. Other researchers have also seen the connection between Maslow's hierarchy and burnout but relate the two in different ways. Shapiro and colleagues used the hierarchy to help healthcare organizations prioritize their interventions logically [69].

The Areas of Worklife (AW) Model of Burnout [70] shows how various imbalances in an employee's worklife can lead to burnout, producing a whole host of negative outcomes, such as absenteeism, poor work quality, reduced patient satisfaction, increased costs, and employee illness, that no employer or employee wants. When an employee's workload is balanced and there is a quality sense of control, community, reward, values, and fairness the employee is likely to remain engaged and enthusiastic in their career. You can see the correlation between the AW Model and Maslow's hierarchy.

Another model, the Job Demands-Resources (JD-R) Model, maintains that when someone has a higher level of job demands than they have adequate resources to address them, burnout can occur [71].

In the Conservation of Resources model, it is believed that burnout results when there are three conditions involving resources, either threats to an individual's ability to derive or maintain resources, a loss of resources, or a lack of return on the use of those resources [72].

When I consider different resources that safeguard against burnout, they all fit neatly into one of Maslow's five levels. You and I all have a need for both self esteem and recognition (esteem from others). We want quality professional relationships and social support (belongingness), a safe environment free from violence in any form whether verbal or physical (safety needs), a balanced life with adequate time for food, water, sleep, and homeostasis (physiological needs), and ultimately the desire for meaning or purpose in work (self-actualization). Deficiencies at any one level may impact burnout to differing extents for individuals but meeting these various needs will keep the risk of burnout low.

Levels of Severity

People experience burnout with various degrees of severity. One person's experience can be mild or almost unnoticeable, whereas another person's experience could be severe and devastatingly obvious. Bearing this in mind, there is no one-size-fits-all solution because burnout results from complex interactions of each unique work system with very unique personalities. Understanding common contributors to burnout can effectively shift our focus from treatment to prevention.

I have personally read several books and articles by health professionals reducing the solution to burnout as solely individual in nature. One author used a humorous analogy that a physician with burnout avoids healthy personal choices, like someone choosing to avoid washing the dishes when they pile up in the sink or failing to maintain a vehicle. Condescension and assumptions aside, in reality, studies paint a different picture – that while there are benefits to individual-focused strategies, they do not fully address or resolve overall clinician burnout [73].

I have concluded that focusing only on personal solutions as a cure-all to solve burnout is akin to placing a bandage over a flesh-eating ulcer. Self-care can only accomplish so much in a system that is riddled with toxic environments that are ignored, and therefore continue to pressure and prevent workers from having the option of personal healthy choices. When the air in a coal mine is toxic, there is little that a miner can do except try and escape it.

Telling someone suffering from burnout to simply *"get more sleep"* fails to consider the underlying and systemic factors that can prevent a person from sleeping in the first place! Insomnia can actually be a result of burnout syndrome, not just a contributing factor. Other external factors may also prevent health professionals from sleeping, such as calls at night/ early morning regarding ailing patients, the stress from increasing amounts of administrative tasks and paperwork infiltrating their home life. "Get more sleep" discredits or minimizes the cause of burnout, doing more harm than good by further propagating the myth that burnout is mainly the result of poor individual choices. It is a wholly atomistic view of the human experience, ignoring important contexts of the healthcare profession and culture.

> **FOCUSING ONLY ON PERSONAL SOLUTIONS AS A CURE-ALL TO SOLVE BURNOUT IS AKIN TO PLACING A BANDAGE OVER A FLESH-EATING ULCER.**

Healthcare Culture—Stoicism

Speaking of the healthcare culture, society especially expects certain *good* or *hardworking* characteristics to be overemphasized to an unhealthy level in our profession. Indeed, actions such as never stopping for a break, working through lunch hours, or always being present in the office, clinic, or ward may not be praised but is often expected. The healthcare environment is emotionally taxing as a result of high stress situations. Meeting one's physiological and safety needs is invaluable in navigating a stressful environment and maintaining a mentality conducive to the highest performance. The importance of this cannot be overstated, as it is not only significant to the individual but also to the patient to ensure safe patient care, reduced medical errors and the best possible patient outcomes. In a high stress environment, taking breaks to recharge physically and mentally should be mandatory, and seen as commonplace.

Imagine an attending or resident physician who has to complete inpatient hospital rounds on 15+ seriously ill patients and then immediately after rounds, meets a full outpatient clinic of 20+ patients (using minimal estimates). This often occurs without a break in between, which means likely an entire day without eating a meal or drinking sufficient fluid. In such cases, physiological needs are not met.

In one UK study, researchers compared the hydration and urine output of the critically ill patients in the intensive care unit (ICU) to that of the junior doctors/physician trainees taking care of them. Shockingly, urine output was so insufficient that for 22 percent of the days, the physicians studied were at risk of acute kidney injury and 1 percent of the time they were considered to actually have acute kidney injury [74]. These same physicians were twice as likely as their patients to have oliguria, which is when the urine output drops dangerously low for 6 hours or more. You can probably (and unsurprisingly) guess that this study called for healthcare organizations to improve access to water fountains!

In another scenario, a physician arrived at the clinic late; they had been *preoccupied* supporting the family members of one of their acutely ill or dying patients on the hospital ward. The physician's patients and the clinic staff members will not likely understand these unexpected events, delays, and added stressors that caused the physician to be late. It is not difficult to imagine conflict with staff or patients over their late arrival or even verbal abuses targeting their character. Now, the physician has lost the opportunity to experience an understanding relational culture that brings that sense of 'belonging' Maslow talked about. This impacts esteem and a sense of safety. Unfortunately, these kinds of situations are commonplace in the field of healthcare. It is unlikely that the clinician will explain why they were late, whether that's due to time constraints, patient confidentiality, or the stigma of *making excuses* for it. It is possible they will conduct their clinic hamstrung by their physical and emotional state even if unknown to them.

Heroes versus Superheroes during COVID-19

There is a rather huge distinction between the due recognition of heroes for their self-sacrifice and hard work helping others, and the dynamic that takes place when society ignores or justifies the inhumane conditions or treatment of those persons under the camouflage of *superhero status*. During the COVID-19 pandemic, stories and photos of healthcare professionals portrayed this grim reality, with stories of workers speaking out against the lack of personal protective equipment, and photos of workers curled into a fetal position on a supply shelf just to find a place for some much-needed rest. These are the *superheroes* who were also sleeping on the hospital floor while executive offices lay empty after 5 pm. Healthcare workers were denied the basic physiological needs within Maslow's hierarchy for adequate sleep – let alone any other fundamental need.

We heard stories in the United States of healthcare professionals being denied their basic need for safety, and even threatened or fired for speaking out against such injustices as the lack of personal protective equipment. Some organizations denied food donations intended for healthcare professionals to their respective facilities. I personally read reports of housing and apartment managers leaving notes for healthcare workers saying that they would no longer be welcome to live there because of their close proximity to those with COVID-19, a discrimination and another denial based solely on their occupation. What do you do for someone that you consider a hero? Would you fight for their rights to basic human needs? The widespread burnout and mistreatment of healthcare professionals existed before the pandemic, but it may have reached a critical point during it, further affecting the overall stability of the healthcare system, and these will no doubt continue after the pandemic panic subsides.

Normalcy of Inhumanity

Those who pursue a healthcare career usually do so with an important understanding of the extreme demands of the career and the ongoing expectation and pressure to place the needs of others before their own. However, the manner in which this occurs, and the degree of inhumanity displayed towards healthcare professionals is not something that should be expected or ever referred to as normal. The society that utilizes the healthcare system or those running healthcare organizations, must be aware that healthcare professionals, including physicians, are not the superhumans that some may wish to see them as. They too have limiting fundamental needs, and consideration of their needs as a fellow human, with a display of empathy will always be warranted.

Beck and Call

There is a common misconception that clinicians should always be available. Staff are praised for answering calls in the middle of the night or returning to the office on a non-emergent whim. When a clinician speaks out against non-emergent calls, or delays their response to a routine request, then they are labeled 'difficult' or described as 'uncaring'. Isn't it right to have time off or make an attempt at uninterrupted sleep?

Fractured sleep and insomnia already plague the health profession; time away from work should be protected.

With consideration, it's not difficult to make a distinction between urgent, emergent, and routine queries before making a call. Expectations on our healthcare professionals should not be based on impatience or convenience. Clinicians either must speak out against being hit with routine calls off shift or risk continuing to propagate the notion that they are always available. In the latter case, they will show up to write a routine prescription or stay late to do so, possibly just to avoid any potential conflict. They may also begin to believe that this behavior is the norm depending on the stage their career is at. Comply once or twice, and soon it will become an expectation, a normal occurrence for staff to continue their demands. It may not be intentionally intrusive, because they just assume that "Dr. ___ doesn't mind, since they did it the last time" or "Dr. ___ is on call so I should just page him with this routine request." The cycle will continue until the clinician either speaks out or burns out, becoming cynical and exhausted; meanwhile the patients are put at greater risk. The longer that it takes to speak out about a concern, the more difficult it may be for others to understand why such inevitable protest eventually occurs.

Every healthcare professional is a human-being with personal responsibilities to themselves and those who are in their personal circle of responsibility, and not only to their 'career', to their 'patient population', 'clinic', or 'co-workers'. Taking a break, a holiday, or simply time for nutrition or to sleep uninterrupted is not a symptom of selfish entitlement. In any occupation, we all need to be able to clock-out at the end of the day and not take work home with us.

Of course, clinicians might be assigned to be on-call, but that certainly doesn't exempt them from empathetic consideration. All calls should be triaged prior to being placed, and at critical hours of the day, when one would likely be asleep, queries that are non-urgent should be channeled to the employee at less critical times of day. If staff are unsure how to triage calls, policies can be put into place and training provided on how to do so safely.

Importantly, to what extent are healthcare professionals expected to place their patients before their own health needs, if in so doing they harm themselves and inadvertently the patients as well? Is this not in breach of the Hippocratic oath upon which the core tenets of modern healthcare were founded? When the health of health-care personnel suffers due to occupational stressors, patients suffer as a result. As a society we should respect each other's time and autonomy. Patient and clinician safety require it!

THE LONGER THAT IT TAKES TO SPEAK OUT ABOUT A CONCERN, THE MORE DIFFICULT IT MAY BE FOR OTHERS TO UNDERSTAND WHY SUCH INEVITABLE PROTEST EVENTUALLY OCCURS.

Until 2014, it seemed that healthcare worker well-being was left out of the equation to the success of the healthcare system, and performance measures were termed as the "triple aim" [75]. The goal of the triple aim was to improve patient care, enhance the health of the population, and reduce costs. It's difficult to achieve those goals if they often come at the expense of healthcare workers! In 2014, the phrase "quadruple aim" was put forth and included additional measures to improve the work life of healthcare personnel [76]. I agree wholeheartedly with the researchers who propose that this added goal should in fact be prioritized as a key measure of organizational performance [77]. The other three goals hang on the success of reaching this fourth aim, and likely each of the other performance goals will be obtained easier and quicker with a united and engaged workforce.

The Norm of Overtime

To talk about the respect of time and autonomy, we must tackle the issue of *overtime*. Within the National Health Service (NHS) in England, 55.9 percent of staff in 2019 reported working extra unpaid hours each week [78]. More than 60 percent of staff working in the community and in mental health/learning disability reported working additional unpaid hours. Extra time should be compensated, yet it has become a normal occurrence and perhaps an expectation within healthcare, that these extra hours are not compensated. Respecting staff time with pay demonstrates that they are valued in their work and gives them a deserved sense of reward for providing a needed service by their organization and its patients.

The Little Spoken Yet Large Toll of Abuse and Violence on Burnout

Violence against healthcare professionals is the "hush, hush" secret few talk about, and even fewer know about, but it is a very tangible contributor to clinician burnout. The relationship between healthcare professionals and patients denotes such a critical factor that can affect burnout. A good relationship is protective, so when that sense of protection is broken by physical or psychological abuse, the effect on burnout is significant [79].

The tragic and gruesome murder of a family physician in Canada captured public attention. The news described that a patient entered the clinic of the physician with a hammer and machete. Of course, this kind of scenario is not very common, however what is more common are acts of verbal and physical abuse which occur at the hands of patients or patient visitors every day. These don't reach the public ear, and it's questionable whether reporting them would lead to changes at all [80]. The gruesome murder story was published, and the community was shocked.

> **VIOLENCE AGAINST HEALTHCARE PROFESSIONALS IS THE "HUSH, HUSH" SECRET FEW TALK ABOUT, AND EVEN FEWER KNOW ABOUT, BUT IT IS A VERY TANGIBLE CONTRIBUTOR TO CLINICIAN BURNOUT.**

Is there blame to be placed beyond the perpetrator, and if so, where? To that question, some commented on the physician's treatment of his patients. Though the question evoked speculation of whether this patient was mistreated by the physician who was killed, but would the answer to that question somehow make this killing more justifiable? Nothing could ever justify such brutality. Some people wondered if the patient was drug seeking and demanded drugs which the physician refused. Yes, this scenario could lead to a very uncomfortable and potentially dangerous scenario. The motives to the murder are still unknown. Aside from people blaming the victim, is there any blame for the system? Did the organizational system, or in fact healthcare training, prepare this physician to deal with conflict?

Some physicians are taught how to de-escalate conflicts, though training of this nature is not uniform. All physicians and healthcare professionals should be provided formal conflict training; imagine the added internal confidence a professional would have if trained by professionals from disciplines more accustomed to navigating high tension conflicts. Conflict resolution or de-escalation should be mandated as a part of the medical, nursing, or other healthcare personnel curriculum. In healthcare, a highly relational discipline, conflict is inevitable.

A study in China which surveyed 1,656 physicians from various specialties in 123 public hospitals, reported that violence was common on the job, whether it was verbal abuse (nearly 93 percent), physical threats (88 percent) or physical assault (81 percent). Each of these forms of abuse resulted in lower job satisfaction, emotional exhaustion, and some physicians intending to leave their positions prematurely [81]. Verbal abuse was most common and had the largest impact on emotional exhaustion and decreased job satisfaction. Verbal abuse and threats of abuse increased the motivation of physicians to leave the front-line, and those who had the misfortune of experiencing physical abuse intended to quit their medical practice completely and indefinitely [82].

A study of 2,397 nurses in Australia found that over half of them had experienced violence on the job, and those who did, demonstrated higher rates of burnout [83]. The prevalence of workplace violence globally ranges from 50 percent to 88 percent [84]. Workplace violence towards healthcare workers is also an issue in the US. In 2012, the National Institute for Occupational Safety and Health (NIOSH) created the Occupational Health Safety Network (OHSN) a voluntary system where hospitals could submit data on occupational injury to staff members. This network was decommissioned in September 2019 according to the NIOSH website [85]. From 2012 to the end of 2015, there were 116 facilities that provided pertinent data. Injuries commonly occurred from violence against female staff (66 percent). Worker injuries also happened on in-patient adult wards (29 percent), in the outpatient emergency departments (19 percent), in critical care units (7.4 percent) and on behavioral health or psychiatric wards (6.8 percent) [86].

Forty-eight percent of those violent events resulted in lost days of work, job restrictions or transfers. Very much a concern, violence incidence rates among the hospitals in that network increased on average 23 percent per year from 2012 to 2015. The data found that the largest reporting groups of violent incidents were nurses and nursing assistants, possibly due to the larger amount of time that nursing staff spend with the patient in proportion to other staff groups. I'm uncertain as to why there is a lack of reporting from physicians on the incidence of violence against them, but many studies in the US have shown a high risk of workplace violence against physicians in psychiatry, emergency medicine, and general practice [87].

Employees in another study mentioned an unspoken attitude that violence is an expected aspect of their work and when it occurred, it was rationalized and normalized [88].

The important thing from this discussion is that not only is the rate of violent events critical, but records should also account for verbal abuse, which occurs more often and underreported, as noted in the study by Shi et al.

Other studies have also noted gender differences in abused staff, with higher rates of abuse reported by female healthcare professionals. An analysis of 14 studies from multiple countries including Great Britain, USA, Israel, Portugal, Italy, Spain, Australia, Canada, Germany and Hong Kong among others, found that female nurses were more likely to be verbally abused and male nurses to be physically abused [89]. Studies in Italy and Japan found similar results [90]. In China and Norway, they found that males there – whether nurses or physicians – were likely to experience greater verbal and physical violence than females [91]. In a Norway study that followed physicians for 20 years after graduating medical school, there was a clear correlation of higher workplace violence against young physicians earlier in their career and those working in psychiatry [92].

Not only is violence a contributing factor for burnout, but it is also a risk for the development of post-traumatic stress disorder and psychological illness [93]. I cannot understate the importance of reporting and mitigating violence against our healthcare professionals.

Violence Prevention

In British Columbia Canada (BC), statistics in 2015 showed that nurses accounted for an astonishing 31 percent of the occupational injuries due to violence [94]. This exceeded injuries to personnel in security and law enforcement, who accounted for only 14 percent of violent workplace incidents. In 2019, the healthcare and social services sector accounted for the majority of workplace violence injury claims (59 percent) [95].

The US Bureau of Labor Statistics reported in 2018 that 73 percent of workers in the private industry who experienced workplace violence, were in the healthcare and social assistance sector [96]. The majority of them were women and required at least 31 days off of work for recovery.

An interesting study compared medical-surgical and mental health specialties in BC as well as the type of violence prevention training that they received. Greater than 90 percent of nurses completed mandatory education on violence prevention [97], though the strategies against violence varied between organizations across BC. The passive forms of education, usually conducted online, were found not to help nurses feel safe at work. What did contribute to feelings of safety? Interestingly, it was active simulations/drills and patient tailored care plans, with input from nursing staff, to help deal with patients who were at high risk for aggression, that was more reassuring to nurses.

Overall, nurses felt less safe when they were expected to intervene in violent cases, and when working on units without fixed alarm devices [98]. Workers felt strongly that the personal support of managers/supervisors is critical in alleviating the psychological impact of workplace violence [99].

Violence is a critical and growing concern within the healthcare system. Organizations need to step up and enforce zero tolerance for all forms of violence, physical or verbal. Managers and administrators should be intentional about providing an atmosphere where staff are comfortable and encouraged to report abuse; each report, then must be taken seriously and investigated with the appropriate follow up, which communicates to your personnel that you value them highly! Strict and enforceable repercussions need to be established at the policy level to deal with abusers. Careful thought should be used to develop preventative and protective strategies. Active education through simulation or drills seems to be much more effective than passive instruction.

In summary, contributors to burnout are multifactorial; however, there are many areas that can be improved within the organizational system to aim for prevention!

Key Chapter Points

- Physicians in early stage/mid-career of practice may be at a higher risk of burnout.

- Review *Maslow's Hierarchy of Needs* as a tool to insightfully understand burnout.

- Conceptual models explain how burnout occurs, A-W model, JD-R model, and the Conservation of Resources model.

- Severity of burnout should be thought of on a continuum, so there is no one size fits all solution. Prevention is key.

- Health culture stoicism, normalcy of inhumanity, expected overtime and under-appreciation contribute to increased risk of burnout.

- Enforce zero tolerance for all forms of violence and abuse. Establish and uphold consequences for perpetrators to safeguard our healthcare personnel.

- Encourage all personnel to report verbal and physical violence and each report should be investigated with actionable outcomes and repercussions.

- Educate personnel through simulation or active learning in conflict resolution.

CHAPTER 5:
RACIAL AND ETHNIC BIAS

"I heard that the resident, the young

black girl, isn't doing so well."

Goals: Educate on implicit bias to promote equality.

Each of us can easily carry implicit or unconscious biases within us, whether it is toward a person or group of people; these biases exist in every career discipline. Biases could be related to gender, ethnic/racial, or even based on physical features etc. Biases can also be explicit (conscious and controllable forms of bias). An example of a bias that existed for many years was that men had careers and women only stayed home to look after families. This bias still exists today, whether it is held by someone consciously or unconsciously, as a product of their environment or situational upbringing. Ethnic/racial bias is also common.

Look at the quote heading this chapter. What would be the motive for using the woman's skin color in relation to the comment that was made between program coordinators about performance? This biased statement was likely made unconsciously.

Women physicians were uncommon in the medical field at one time, and it is still uncommon to see black women who are physicians. In the United States in 2018, black physicians regardless of gender, made up only 5 percent of all active physicians [100]. In 2007, the Association of Faculties of Medicine of Canada began a voluntary national survey of medical students, which included questions relating to ethnicity and socioeconomic backgrounds, which had not been collected in previous years. Response rates were low, but from these statistics, only 2.9 percent of medical students identified as black [101].

As seen in the chapter quote, the existence of bias came to light when a statement was made that distinguished or categorized another person based on obscure characteristics, such as their gender or ethnic background. I can imagine that if someone were to change that statement to read the 'young white girl,' it would be unlikely that the hearer would know who they are talking about because the demographic is saturated with people that fit that description. That would be even more true if someone was to say the 'young white guy'.

Why is it that visible minority groups are often described by their cultural group/ethnicity/race whereas a 'majority group' is not? Regardless of whether the bias is conscious or unconscious, greater awareness is needed to understand that these biases exist and can result in harmful stereotypes and even more harmful consequences of these stereotypes. The dictionary puts it perfectly, defining a stereotype as "something conforming to a fixed or general pattern. Especially a standardized mental picture…that represents an oversimplified opinion, prejudiced attitude, or uncritical judgment" [102]. Let's examine our lives for the presence of stereotypes and tainted viewpoints. When one is aware of potential bias we can reflect and be more conscientious about how it influences our actions.

The Influence of Bias in Hiring

Biases may also influence actions. An executive deciding on staff to consider for hire can be led by implicit or explicit bias. When all other aspects of an application are held the same, one study showed that applicants with ethnic names are less likely to be hired for the same position as someone with a common or less ethnically distinct name [103]. Unless people openly discuss and acknowledge their conscious or unconscious biases, then this issue will continue into the future of healthcare.

Implicit Bias

A lab at Harvard University has conducted research into bias and attempted to create a tool to help discover a person's bias via a series of online questionnaires and experiments [104]. These tools are one attempt to shed light onto this issue and create awareness; another method is self-reflection and conscious awareness. Within the workplace, biases should be addressed proactively, and not solely in reaction to a discriminatory event. Organizations should provide education to staff on diversity, equity, and inclusion, making no assumptions that each staff member is of the same understanding when it comes to values, and being respectful or considerate of diverse co-workers. The organization has a duty to clearly convey and demonstrate their values and attitudes to every staff member. This training effort not only aligns all staff to a shared understanding of how the organization views diversity, equity, and inclusion, but also cultivates a healthy environment wherein staff members can better hold themselves and each other accountable when issues arise that don't align with the values set forth by the organization.

WITHIN THE WORKPLACE, BIASES SHOULD BE ADDRESSED PROACTIVELY, AND NOT SOLELY IN REACTION TO A DISCRIMINATORY EVENT.

How Bias Relates to Burnout

Considering the Areas of Worklife model (Section 2, Chapter 1) in relating the issue of bias to burnout development, you can see that when company values and worker values misalign, burnout can develop. For example, if a company does not demonstrate that a diverse and inclusive employee base is among their values, then those who are of a diverse cultural background will feel the tension of this misalignment of values. Organizations need to take action not only by stating their values and commitments in writing but demonstrating their commitment by ensuring diversity and inclusiveness among their employees. Each employee should feel respected, valued as a team member, and free from discrimination. If those at fault for discrimination in the workplace are not held accountable, then it will be apparent that the organization does not live up to its word. Employees most affected by this hypocrisy will be at high risk for burnout.

Key Chapter Points

- People should openly discuss and strive to become aware of their conscious or unconscious biases.
- When one is aware of their biases they can reflect, become conscientious, and considerate in the way they refer to others.
- The organization should provide education to staff on diversity, equity, and inclusion, clearly conveying and demonstrating their values.
- When company values and worker values misalign then burnout can develop.

Try the Implicit Bias tool

CHAPTER 6:
GENDER BIAS

*"That doctor is always pulling the feminist
card. She's overdoing it now."*

Goals: Educate on gender bias to promote gender equality.

It's important to be cognizant of gender biases and in doing so, mitigate any discrimination that occurs as a result. A female physician spoke up during the hiring process for a new staff physician about the low number of female staff currently in the department, and the lack of consideration of female candidates applying for the physician job position. Superiors acknowledged her observations and went on to consider more female candidates in the hiring pool.

Soon, malicious talk circulated through the office about the outspoken physician, propagating the phrase that she used up her 'feminist card' quota. A few months later, that same physician applied for a male dominated position as the head of the division. Then, people said she was *striving too much* and *overachieving*. You might be surprised to know that the staff member who made the 'feminist card comments' was a woman. That story alerted me to the fact that gender bias, usually perceived as only by men towards women, can also flow from women who have accepted the limitation that some roles are only suited for men.

Women face the gender bias in healthcare and most career fields. Regardless of how bias-neutral a company presents itself outwardly, staff members can remain biased implicitly or explicitly as seen in these two scenarios. Women who aim to achieve successes are often seen as *over-achieving*, whereas their male counterparts are described with words such as *achievers* or *successful*. Together, our healthcare profession must work to transform that prejudiced thought-culture.

Mitigating Gender Bias

Women may always have to deal with this bias, as people will at times seek division based on the characteristics that make us unique (ethnicity, gender, and so on...). Training workshops and discussions cannot change the hearts of individuals or organizational cultures and systems made up of them.

I'm not implying here that education on gender bias should not occur or isn't important. Women who have been trained to expect some hardship and understand this bias are less likely to be shocked into submission or skulk into the shadows of mediocrity. If when bias rears its ugly head, we're not caught off guard, we can better respond to it. That can be easier said than done without a strategy in place. When discrimination is directed at you, you can tap into the power of the three questions in the resiliency framework discussed in section 1 chapter 1.

Is this an opinion or fact?

Does what they think change the reality of how I see myself?

Do I have anything to prove?

Let's practice applying them again, this time to the statement that 'women are overachieving'. Opinion or fact? Overachiever in the Merriam Webster dictionary means "one who achieves success over and above the standard or expected level especially at an early age" [105]. Since no research has shown achievement levels to be dictated by gender (as those who adopt this bias prefer to assume), you can rightly conclude that this statement is an opinion and not a fact.

To the second question, the comment 'overachiever' in no way changes anything if you firmly believe that gender does not limit your abilities to capably handle your role.

Do you have something to prove to the person conveying that statement? Do you just let your success and achievements speak for you? Maybe, might be the tempting answer. However, if that person is a chronic offender who regularly makes condescending remarks regarding gender, you may want to prove to that person that their remarks are inappropriate, not so much to defend yourself, but presenting an opportunity for the other person to grow and be educated. Proof is "evidence that compels acceptance by the mind of a truth or a fact" [106]. There is no need to stoop to a biased person's level, but go ahead, speak up if needed and show that women can be successful in the work that's been put on their hearts and minds, with hard work and dedication.

Gender Equality in the Healthcare Field

Promoting and enforcing gender equality within the company is key to maintaining a diverse and equitable workforce. If gender bias is systemic, those who discriminate against others are not held accountable and employees will recognize it. When those employees see unfair treatment or disciplinary actions not matching the organization's claims of inclusivity and equitability the potential for burnout skyrockets [107].

Letting your success and achievements speak for you is difficult, if not impossible, when bias is so systemic that those who are discriminated against won't be duly recognized by the company. They will likely work even harder than other employees to prove themselves *worthy* of equivalent promotions or rewards granted employees

THE WORK OVERLOAD TO PROVE YOURSELF WORTHY CAN HAVE SIGNIFICANT EFFECTS ON YOUR HEALTH AND PERSONAL LIFE, LEADING TO BURNOUT.

of the opposite gender. The work overload to prove yourself worthy can have significant effects on your health and personal life, leading to burnout. If the organizations will not stand up against discrimination in support of their employees, the resulting toxic environment will ultimately sacrifice the health of the employees, the organization, and the patients that are cared for.

Key Chapter Points

- Be cognizant of gender bias and in doing so, mitigate any discrimination.
- Use the Resiliency Framework questions when discrimination and gender bias is directed towards you.
- Within healthcare organizations gender equality should be promoted and enforced.

CHAPTER 7:
UNREALISTIC EXPECTATIONS

"I've lost hope in humanity."

Goals: Ensure adequate staffing and coverage. Allay moral distress.

What causes people to lose hope in humanity? How do minor irritations with a few people progress to such a grave and intense emotional issue?

An emergency room physician said the following words to a colleague who called in sick: "Chris must be on his death bed if he's really not going to come in today". Turns out that Chris retracted his sick call and showed up to work. He entered the unit looking weathered and said he had lost hope in humanity. That level of cynicism can surely be a sign and result of burnout.

What was the background that caused him to express that level of despair? In this case, it seemed as though society fell short of his expectations when, as a physician, even he was unable to take a day off due to illness. It was evidence that physicians are held to a higher standard than a non-professional employee; however, you will often notice this double standard when it comes to sick time. Society usually expects that physicians rarely get sick or need time off due to unexpected emergencies whether personal or familial. Some studies have indeed shown that physicians often suffer from less health concerns than the general population [108], likely due to increased insight on the causes of medical disease.

The cynical joke that Chris ought to be on his death bed is actually a reflection of the attitude of many, that a physician should never call in sick. Unfortunately, physicians and healthcare personnel often think the same thing, being acutely aware of the strains that their absence will place on staff and patients. You would think the healthcare field would extend more empathy to someone who is unwell, but too many see a physician's illness or time off as an inconvenience.

On one occasion, a surgeon became suddenly ill, requiring a hospital stay and possible surgery. The first reaction and comments from the administration was how difficult and inconvenient this situation was for them since they would need to reschedule patients. Contrasting that attitude, other surgeons at the hospital stepped up and offered to cover her clinics and see any patients who required urgent appointments.

Administrators should be careful to watch for the issues that unduly contribute to the strain on their physicians. Physicians on contract or working in a private facility may not be afforded the same benefits regarding time off as employees. For those who are employees of a healthcare organization, many physicians who do have vacation and personal/sick time, often say that they cannot use it. This can be due to perceived stigmas on being off, clinical obligations, or impeding moral dilemma. Usually when unused, that time does not carry forward and is lost forever. Of course, each person and the system they work under is different, so the ability to use personal/sick time or vacation time varies between physicians – but I have found these nuances to be true. Those working in a group practice may find it easier to get the appropriate coverage than specialists or private practice physicians.

> **ADMINISTRATORS SHOULD BE CAREFUL TO WATCH FOR THE ISSUES THAT UNDULY CONTRIBUTE TO THE STRAIN.**

Longer Shifts Versus Improved Handovers

We must obtain and preserve a healthy balance between shift length, maintaining continuity of care, and minimizing healthcare errors. Some strongly believe that physicians need to work longer hours and continuous shifts so as not to interrupt the continuity of care; the logic is that this will decrease handovers which could lead to miscommunication and errors. Continuous extended hours, however, can be detrimental to patient safety and clinician well-being.

One US study of four academic hospital intensive care units randomly placed intensive care physicians into groups with either a continuous work schedule of day shifts for 14 consecutive days, or a weekday schedule with weekends covered by colleagues [109]. Of the 1,900 patients in the study, those seen in the continuous work schedule showed higher length of stay and higher, yet not statistically significant, mortality. Furthermore, those physicians who worked in the continuous schedule indicated statistically significant, higher levels of burnout, job distress, and worse work-home life balance than those with weekend coverage [110].

Staffing Shortages Contribute to Burnout

Studies universally show that chronic staff shortages increase risk of burnout for people within nursing, pharmacy, and other healthcare disciplines. In a study with over 10,000 nurses there was a 23 percent greater risk of experiencing emotional exhaustion with each added patient exceeding 4 patients per nurse [111]. The international survey included nurses from two provinces in Canada, Pennsylvania in the US, and England and Scotland in the UK. It was found that nurses in all countries demonstrated high levels of burnout. Those who felt that they had poor organizational support were twice as likely to have high burnout scores. Short-staffed hospitals were rated by nurses as fair or poor with low quality patient care.

Nurses in twelve European countries who completed shifts longer than twelve hours had a much higher likelihood of burnout and job dissatisfaction compared to those who were working 8 hours or less [112]. Staffing shortages often mean longer shifts, to compensate. Over a quarter of the participants in that study worked overtime hours, contributing to their burnout. Pediatric nurses who felt rushed, interrupted, and with their attention constantly divided and stretched thin due to perceived inadequate staffing, suffered increased burnout [113]. Other healthcare professionals may have a similar experience. Unions usually aim to protect nurses and other

STUDIES UNIVERSALLY SHOW THAT CHRONIC STAFF SHORTAGES INCREASE RISK OF BURNOUT FOR PEOPLE WITHIN NURSING, PHARMACY, AND OTHER HEALTHCARE DISCIPLINES.

unionized workers rights to a certain standard; however, these standards are often inadequately applied by organizations and staff shortage continues at the expense of staff and patient well-being. Certainly, some burnout factors are outside of the organization's control; however, focus should be narrowed in on conditions that can be safe guarded, such as working hours, on-call time, and support staff scheduling etc.

It can be difficult to find support staff for physicians when emergent cases present after hours; a physician is expected to stay on shift until that patient is stable whereas their support staff do not. Support staff shift changes still occur regardless, and patient care may be delayed. Healthcare guidelines are not uniform nor offer protection to the entire patient care team. For example, a cardiovascular interventionalist would find it impossible to perform a heart catheterization for a critical patient without the support of multiple staff within the lab, from technicians to nurses. Clinicians can only do as much as they are supported by a team. When a team approach is not maintained, this leads to frustrations and inevitably, burnout.

Moral Distress

Moral distress leads to burnout and applies to healthcare in distinct and unique ways. Moral distress occurs when a physician's ethical values are incongruent with those they are interacting with, whether patients or their family, colleagues, or the health care organization [114]. An example would be when healthcare personnel believe they are being pressured to compromise their ethics by one of those three people or groups mentioned above, and under such circumstances feel unable to change that situation [115]. Healthcare professionals will all be challenged by this scenario at some point within the current system. It is thought to have cumulative effect, where each distressing situation compounds the distress over time with repeated experiences [116].

Burnout from moral distress also occurs in training. Medical students initially show comparable burnout levels to the general college student population until they begin medical school. Prior to medical school and often during medical school, many students will hear satisfying words of encouragement from friends, family, or acquaintances commending them for their hard-work, determination, and ambition to pursue such a noble career in medicine caring for others. However, within the confines of the medical school classroom, and in the hospital during practical experience, they discover that they are then just 'little fish in a big pond'; their attributes, and ambitions are common in the student body and their individual voices are no longer distinct, whether that's a desire to give back to their community, diagnose and heal, or fill a physician need in the developing world. That 'lack of voice' is a serious component in the definition of moral distress. Rarely will hard-work ethic and determination be impressive in medical school where those enrolled are all expected to have these traits as a minimum. It is expected, often without praise or notice unless you get to the very top of the class to receive that recognition.

When this all occurs, the world looks much different to the student; it doesn't seem to value their effort, preparation, or their caring nature which are precisely the attributes the healthcare profession needs. The values healthcare and medical students come into the field with are soon swallowed up by the educational system, or conflict with norms that are portrayed by society. They are seen as *just* another medical student or *just* another resident in a long line of many

MEDICAL STUDENTS INITIALLY SHOW COMPARABLE BURNOUT LEVELS TO THE GENERAL COLLEGE STUDENT POPULATION UNTIL THEY BEGIN MEDICAL SCHOOL.

others with similar goals and qualities. These students lose their individuality, their voice, and possibly their sense of identity. This process is morally distressing to the young student or resident, who might not discuss these feelings or issues with others. They may assume things will get better once they reach the next stage in their training – we all may think that we'll be happier if only we *just* reach that next stage.

For example, a student may cope simply by trying to convince themselves that the conditions and moral distress will improve, and thus they steel themselves up to endure that distress. Similarly, a resident who experiences moral distress may attempt to cope by rationalizing that these issues will subside when they become an attending physician. Surprise! Seniority doesn't grant immunity from moral distress that can affect attending physicians at any stage of their career. The tension may come from different sources as roles evolve, but the challenge remains.

Nurses have also been impacted by moral distress. Indeed, moral distress increases among nurses when they feel powerless, instructed to provide care they judge to be unnecessary, when giving false hope, or if a patient has been 'consented' without being properly informed [117]. One study showed that nurses with 10 or more years of practice had a higher level of moral distress, which the researchers thought was due to a cumulative effect of difficult events that conflicted with their values [118].

Key Chapter Points

- All healthcare personnel should be entitled to time off work.
- Nursing, pharmacy, and other healthcare disciplines experience added stress and increased risk of burnout due to chronic staff shortages or inadequate staffing.
- Moral distress occurs when your ethical values are challenged by the organization, by co-workers in the unit, or by the patient or their family.

CHAPTER 8:
THE STIGMA SURROUNDING MENTAL HEALTH

"Physician, heal thy self."

Goals: Encourage teamwork, normalize seeking help by providing resources, and removing discriminatory measures.

An interesting survey of 567 psychiatrists found that over 15 percent of them had self-prescribed medication for depression in the past, 43 percent of respondents said that they would consider self-medicating for mild or moderate depression, and 7 percent said that they would do so for severe depression [119].

When 43 percent of psychiatrists say that they would self-treat, that means that they would not seek treatment by a physician who could be more objective!

This stands as an eye-opening perspective on the situation among physicians, considering this reluctance particularly by psychiatrists. Based on that data on psychiatrists, I can only imagine the number of physicians in other specialties who may also be self-treating. Some surveys indicate that physicians are unwilling to seek treatment. There are many reasons for this reluctance, and each one should be addressed and remedied in order to provide a culture in which physicians feel comfortable seeking objective help for themselves.

Physicians are not infallible and require great caution against a common misconception that they should be able to diagnose and even 'treat' themselves. I have seen this misconception promoted by utilizing a quoted passage from the Bible "physician, heal thyself", which is found in Luke 4: 23 [120]. What a misuse of that adage, completely out of its correct context. Physicians often bypass their own health and well-being while caring for patients. That's not what Jesus was saying. In the appropriate context, Jesus was in his hometown of Nazareth reading in the temple. There he was asked by the people to perform miracles like he had done in another city, Capernaum. Jesus said this:

"He said to them, "You will surely say this proverb to Me, 'Physician, heal yourself! Whatever we have heard done in Capernaum, do also here in Your country.' Then He said, "Assuredly, I say to you, no prophet is accepted in his own country.""[121]

To paraphrase, He said to the people that often, whatever a prophet does in his own hometown, usually does not change the people's outlook. In that context, He is saying that the most difficult thing would be to 'heal oneself' in order to bring about other's acceptance. In essence, He is stating that healing oneself, performing a miracle, will not lead to the results that the people want.

> IT IS NOT UP TO INDIVIDUAL PHYSICIANS TO MITIGATE THEIR OWN BURNOUT. ON A SOCIETAL LEVEL THE PREVENTION OF BURNOUT WITHIN THE HEALTHCARE FIELD WILL TAKE ALL OF US.

Back to the issue of self-treatment by physicians: it is unlikely that a physician taking matters into their own hands and self-medicating would lead to a positive outcome. External help should be sought to receive objective diagnosis, insight, and a course of action to address health concerns. It is not up to individual physicians to mitigate their own burnout. On a societal level, the prevention of burnout within the healthcare field will take all of us. Organizations need to make changes to address burnout with advice and insight from clinicians so that those changes can directly improve their workflow and patient relations. Healthcare personnel from every discipline need to be involved, as well as affected patients.

Barriers to Help

Granted, there are barriers for physicians when seeking outside help. Clinics may offer appointments for diagnosis and treatment only at times that conflict with physicians' schedules. If you are unable to take time away from work to attend appointments, you are unlikely to find offices with extended hours on nights or weekends. Appointments may also be scarce in disciplines where therapists are in short supply; physicians are less likely to submit to a waitlist [122]. Complicating things further for physicians to obtain help, ironically, one study concluded that 25 percent or more of physicians don't have a primary care doctor [123]. Physicians without a primary care professional to discuss issues with are highly unlikely to receive early intervention, prescription, or referral.

Clinicians might be apprehensive to seeking evaluation and care due to the possibility of receiving any diagnosis that could impact their medical license [124]. Many state medical licensing boards have questions regarding any lifetime history of mental illness [125]. In those cases, a doctor struggling with burnout faces a risk to his or her medical license even though getting that outside help can help them be a healthier and effective physician. Some of those questions from licensing boards are believed to be a violation of the Americans with Disabilities Act (ADA) [126]. The ADA was enacted in 1990 to prevent discrimination against Americans with disabilities [127]. One study found that only 18 medical licensing boards in the US did not have questions in violation of the ADA, which means that 33 did [128].

Protecting the public is a tricky balance. If current regulations deter physicians who could benefit from treatment to avoid it, then more harm is being done than good [129]. Physicians who took an important step to humbly reach out for help and receive treatment where they struggle with burnout or other mental and physical issues ought not be penalized for that decision. There is an important distinction between living with an illness and being impaired by it. Impairment means that there is a functional limitation. The American Medical Association defines impairment as an inability to practice medicine safely and skillfully, whether that be due to a physical or mental illness, natural aging, or substance use [130].

Questionnaires and requests for medical records by some malpractice insurance companies, clinics, and hospitals is discriminatory towards physicians who sought help [131]. Physicians disclosing any past mental health diagnoses could encounter severe changes to their hospital privileges, and to their health or malpractice insurance [132]. In the US, 35 percent of state medical board applications ask whether you ever had a mental health diagnosis, all the way back to childhood and teenage years, yet only 23 percent of those applications inquired about a physical health problem [133]. The American Psychiatric Association and the Federation of State Medical Boards have both indicated that prior history of a mental health issue or substance use does not predict future risks or current impairment [134]. I believe that these credentialing boards should switch their focus from lifetime diagnoses to that of determining current impairment [135].

In nursing, there is a similar scenario, where 30 state licensing boards were found to ask mental health related questions. Twenty-two of them focused on identifying any prior diagnoses without any questions that might help determine current impairment, or applicants were asked inappropriate questions such as to predict their own future impairment [136].

Normalize Seeking Help

Seeking help when needed is exactly what self-aware physicians should do and involves reaching out to others whether it is for consultation, second opinions, assistance, or personal support from outside of patient care. We in healthcare provide safe and effective patient care through a team-based approach with coordinated care between multiple disciplines. The focus in our training, however, often promotes self-sufficiency. The culture that expects physicians to be independent superheroes was evident in a conversation I overheard when healthcare staff were discussing a physician who consulted with colleagues for help. Over the next few days, those staff members became very judgmental of the physician's capabilities, characterizing seeking assistance of other medical specialties as the equivalent of incompetent physician behavior.

We can do better than that to encourage teamwork particularly within healthcare and establish that it is okay to ask for help when needed. That attitude must be fostered during the initial years of education in all healthcare personnel; perhaps if we adjust our attitudes as a whole, we can see supportive attitudes towards healthcare workers improve as a society.

Increasing Transparency and Reducing Stigma

If the human brain is one of the most complex organs in the human body, then why is there such a stigma about 'mental health' when compared to 'physical health'? Discussion about mental health should be widespread and commonplace, like that of physical ailments, free of cultural stigmas.

If we want to encourage physicians and other healthcare workers to seek help with the intense pressures of our profession, instead of deterring them from doing so, then a major overhaul needs to take place in this area. With the many resources, online courses, and educational programs at our disposal, all healthcare personnel can and should have such training as part of their on-boarding procedures. They can be taught signs of depression and risk factors for suicide in order to recognize them in others as well as themselves.

> **IF THE HUMAN BRAIN IS ONE OF THE MOST COMPLEX ORGANS IN THE HUMAN BODY, THEN WHY IS THERE SUCH A STIGMA ABOUT 'MENTAL HEALTH' WHEN COMPARED TO 'PHYSICAL HEALTH'?**

Training programs for physicians, nursing, pharmacy, and other health disciplines should set aside time within the curriculum to provide access to mental health services. Clinics and health networks attached to the training program, with subsidies, would provide easier access and incentives for students and trainees to seek help, particularly if finances are a hindrance. In such a high stress and demanding profession, nothing says "We are supporting you" more than investing in your lives, especially if organizations make available routine screening questionnaires to indicate burnout and psychological distress. These tools help healthcare personnel become more self-aware; the collective information can be anonymized and provided to the organization collectively to assess how they are preforming overall in the support of their staff and personnel. Using measures such as the *Areas of Worklife* tool, common areas of dissatisfaction among staff can help caring employers direct their interventions most effectively [137]. By using screening to reveal burnout and psychological distress, organizational progress can be better measured.

Key Chapter Points

- Normalize seeking help by providing accessible resources for psychological well-being.
- Train staff to recognize signs of depression and signs of burnout.
- Encourage and normalize teamwork.
- Remove discriminatory measures within licensing boards.

Access resources for well-being

SECTION 3:

Individual Factors that Contribute to Burnout

Burnout is an occupational syndrome that presents itself with many contributing factors from the organization. However, there are some individual factors that have been found to impact burnout. Your personality, coping methods, and finances are all factors that can influence burnout. Recognizing these factors can allow us to either change our perspectives for the better – or seek help early when we are at a greater risk.

CHAPTER 9:
PERSONALITY

"He had horrible bedside manner; if he doesn't want to be a doctor he should leave."

Goals: Educate on hazards of the work environment and build awareness of personality traits and personal risk factors.

People who decide on a career in healthcare often enter with the ideals of helping others; healthcare professionals are prepared to give of themselves, including their knowledge, skills, and time, to care for others and in however small a way, they aim to make their communities a better place by alleviating the suffering of the sick.

The warning I received days before classes began, "it only gets worse", was a phrase that renounced the naivety and triggered the contemplation that there was going to be more to this career than I assumed; every student should hear a phrase such as this.

The same is true of many 'helping professions' such as social work, education, psychology, and ministry for example. Indeed, being effective in these careers won't simply be an idealistic outcome of intense studying and achieving high exam scores. Nor will it be just a matter of 'helping others.' Once the rose-tinted glasses come off, it will become evident that many factors make the healthcare profession unpredictable, particularly for physicians. Those who enter know that it will be hard work, but most simply think that it can be overcome by self-effort, whether that equates to studying, reviewing, or preparing. This is not always the case.

Those people who focus and succeed in school often have an internal locus of control over challenging situations [138]. Resilient individuals have this internal locus of control and therefore are highly optimistic that they can succeed. However, you must be able to distinguish that which is outside of your control. The ability to relinquish your attempts to control something that is outside of your control is also a quality of resilient individuals [139].

Attitude is of critical importance to physical and psychological wellbeing, academics, work, and relationships. Two specific attitudes or mindsets will affect each of these aspects of life. One is referred to as a *fixed mindset*, where the person believes that their qualities or identity have been established and developed but are no longer able to be improved or changed. The opposite attitude is called a growth mindset [140]. People with a fixed mindset tend to avoid challenging scenarios and demonstrate low resilience when adversity occurs [141]. They are apprehensive and fearful of demonstrating a lack of intelligence or ability. Those with a growth mindset see learning opportunities in every challenge, and adversities are interpreted as a means to learn and develop.

In the context of medical training, no one formally prepares personnel for what lies outside of their control – life after the classroom. Burnout can strike a person at any point in their career or study, whenever the positives of their occupation erode and the resources to combat the increasing demands diminish. Burnout is the result of multiple factors: personality and resilience, the culture of the organization, and the work environment [142]. Each of these factors and their relation to burnout will be discussed; within this chapter we will look at the personal factors.

Communication

We begin training for whatever career we decide upon as eager students, but psychologically ill prepared to eventually move from student to competent in the field. To make that transition requires gaining a level of competency and becoming psychologically prepared for the workforce. Most times, the environmental or psychological hazards of the medical career are not taught to us as naive students. What does the job really entail? Are there particular hazards, prejudices, things that are commonly faced?

Healthcare is a career field with an environment filled with hazards. Of course, there are hazards associated with ill patients or possible communicable diseases, but it is also a field heavily dependent on good communication; being unprepared to succeed at communicating effectively can be disastrous.

In healthcare, you will interact in a multidisciplinary manner with people different from you in many respects, whether culturally, ethnically, experientially etc. When you study to become a healthcare professional, it's easy to place a lot of mental emphasis on your individual performance. But when you graduate as a medical doctor, for example, you will have to learn rather quickly how to assert yourself and communicate effectively in a community which requires cooperation. Poor communication will stress you, your whole team, and put patients at risk.

As a student, you learned to respond when called upon or provide a calculated presentation, and then within a day you are no longer a medical student but a graduate and expected to communicate well with other members of the team. Some medical school graduates will develop a good communication style with ease. Perhaps they were eager and observant as a student during clinical training, *if they had good examples to go off, that is.*

While some schools have requirements for behavioral sciences training, they only superficially touch on what will be necessary in the real world to navigate day-to-day interactions. Very few healthcare professionals have received formal training on communication. If we are here to 'help people,' how is it that the healthcare workforce receives little of this teaching when most, if not all patient outcomes, are dependent on effective communication and teamwork? We are never taught to expect the 'unexpected' which we soon find out in day-to-day life is more of the norm. Training in conflict resolution will be just as applicable in your life as the details you learned about human physiology because conflicts between nurses, patients, colleagues, and administrators will occur. With training in effective communication, perhaps fewer conflicts would result. How do you successfully work in a team when most of your prior training emphasized individual efforts and competition, such as who would claim the coveted medical or nursing school dean's list positions?

If a physician prescribes a medication or suggests a lifestyle change, think about the partnership that is needed between the two to ensure common understanding. Only if the patient is in agreement will they take the medications or adapt to the lifestyle change your medical training led you to prescribe. Great communication skill is required for that agreement. As can be seen in the quote in the chapter heading, this patient found their physician's level of communication so lacking that they even questioned their interest in their medical practice!

Resilience and Coping

I've heard many commencement speeches inspiring a particular personal attribute called resilience, yet I find that few understand what it actually means to be resilient or how to achieve it. I cannot recall ever having a lesson in school about this rather elusive term or skill. The stories that receive attention regarding resilience are the ones discussing, how someone, regardless of their situation, physical or mental condition, pressed on and overcame barriers or hardships.

Is that all that it means to be resilient? The Merriam-Webster dictionary defines resilience as, 'an ability to recover from or adjust easily to misfortune or change'[143]. Students realize that they need the ability to recover or adjust to change and misfortune but receive little insight into the personal resources needed and how to develop their resilience.

In our field of healthcare, with its high risk of burnout, resilience is a powerful help. What components influence resilience, what steps can be taken to increase it, and what tools are available to become skilled at making these life adjustments successfully? Kumpfer's theoretical model describes 6 important areas that influence resilience: the actual challenge or stressor itself, the environment, the individual's personalities, the outcome, the way that the individual interacts with the environment, and how they interact with the outcomes. In summary, the level of perceived challenge or stress is affected by how the person interprets these challenges or stress. You can use techniques such as reframing, active coping, or changing environments to influence how your environment impacts you. Within the environment, there is a balance required between stressors and protective aspects such as family, culture, colleagues, and work/school.

There are at least 5 internal factors that influence your resilience: your emotional, behavioral, physical, cognitive, and spiritual makeup (See image). You can develop each one of these areas. In professional discussions on resilience, much has been said about promoting balance in the personal and work life. This holds relevance to the topic of burnout in healthcare careers. Consistently, these writers and speakers emphasize the importance for employees to increase activities that hold deep personal interest or enjoyment, and the benefit of learning and using various proven stress coping techniques. As seen in the framework below, there are many things which can influence resilience.

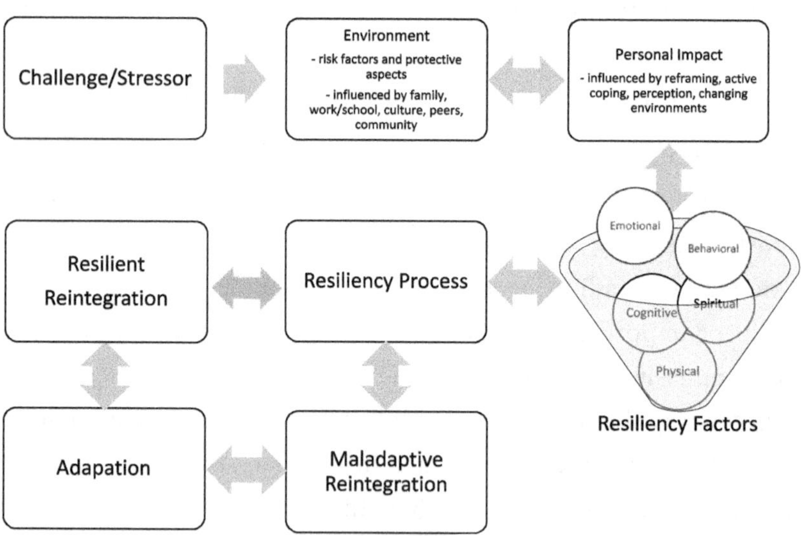

When misfortune or change occurs, the misfortune is generally portrayed as something that is external and needs to be dealt with, such as a family hardship, financial burden, or career crisis. However, what's important is the internal way you perceive and respond to the change or misfortune.

Are physicians lacking resilience? No, in fact, one study found that physicians demonstrate a higher level of resilience or adaptability than the general working population [144]. Researchers measured resilience by using a questionnaire to survey 30,000 physicians, of which 5,445 responded. Those

with higher resilience also had less overall burnout, depersonalization, and emotional exhaustion. Still, 29 percent of physicians with high resilience scores still had symptoms of burnout. Thus, increasing resilience alone will not solve the issue of burnout.

Conscientious, Perfectionist, and Burned Out

Your personality traits are determined by multiple interactions of the environment, genes, and combinations of each [145]. Trainers in sport or academics often tell us that our success will be determined by our effort, and that 'how much we put in, is how much we will get out,' again, the internal locus of control [146].

Is that a realistic view of the world? In medicine, we spend a minimum of 8 years of education having that statement engrained in our minds. It is outside of the classroom, that we so often discover that there is nothing that even the most astute physician can do to prevent a negative diagnosis or change a negative environment or situation. We must therefore distinguish and demarcate what the uncontrollable aspects of life are.

When faced with a negative situation, personal perceptions matter. Successful adaptation to a negative environment is more likely if you can maintain the confidence that you can make a difference and modify the circumstances by action or seek help from others [147]. This may be difficult for students in healthcare professions, where the training is very competitive and individualistic. Students are taught early on that success is a result of their actions, which then assumes that any negativity or lack of success is a direct reflection of their personal actions or inabilities. Self-blame has serious, depressing, and detrimental psychological consequences. Conscientious people (caring deeply about socially prescribed norms, control, and planning) have a higher risk of burnout, sometimes accentuated by perfectionism and great expectations on themselves [148]. Others with neurotic tendencies have risk of burnout, as they usually find any frustrating experiences to be overwhelming. Their reactions to them may be feelings of anger, hostility, anxiety, guilt and depression [149]. In the general population, neuroticism is associated with increased risk for depression, post-traumatic stress disorder (PTSD), and suicidal ideation [150].

Perfectionism can be evident in people striving for perfection and pursuing a high standard, or in those who manifest this tendency fearing criticism, imperfection, or making mistakes. This is termed as perfectionistic striving or perfectionistic concern respectively [151]. Children and adolescents show evidence of perfectionism by an unhealthy need for recognition and acceptance from others, and a belief that their self-worth is determined by their proximity to perfection [152]. Perfectionists of all ages can display compulsiveness and sensitivity to mistakes. Some even believe that

> **CONSCIENTIOUS PEOPLE (CARING DEEPLY ABOUT SOCIALLY PRESCRIBED NORMS, CONTROL, AND PLANNING) HAVE A HIGHER RISK OF BURNOUT, SOMETIMES ACCENTUATED BY PERFECTIONISM AND GREAT EXPECTATIONS ON THEMSELVES.**

others mandate perfection from them. Flett and Hewitt described in their article, how many perfectionists usually don't seek help due to self-consciousness and unwillingness to disclose imperfection. They also have higher tendencies to harm themselves and have suicidal ideation [153]. In another analysis by Hill and Curran, they found that perfectionistic concern (fearing criticism, imperfection, or making mistakes) was associated with burnout.

A person who is conscientious and driven by perfectionism is often viewed in the corporate world as a person with good work ethics, strong motivation, and successful. Within the healthcare field and educational system, leaders often give a priority to applicants with these traits over other applicants.

Now, I'm not trying to label certain personality traits as good or bad, but simply discussing them in the context of burnout. Organizations should support those people who may be at greater risk, and our health-care personnel need to be self-aware and comfortable to seek help early. A number of studies have seen a connection between personality traits and struggles with psychological distress, depression, and anxiety among those in the health care profession.

Another personality trait identified by psychologists is 'reality weakness' which involves troublesome thoughts that border between fantasy and reality, and difficulty with identity, self-direction, and trusting others [154]. The presence of this trait is associated with severe depression, suicidal ideation, and a low likelihood of obtaining help [155]. Dr. Tyssen has also found that being of young age increased the risk for severe depression by 10 percent, reality weakness doubled it, and neuroticism tripled it [156]! A high-risk combination! And those extroverts? There were few that reported depression symptoms; being extrovert seemed to protect against symptoms of burnout.

Anyone in any career could be at a mental health risk, lose hope and career satisfaction, burn out, and suffer depression. Should we be including an additional subject in education, especially healthcare training, that teaches about personality traits, gives an accurate picture of the career environment, and includes practical skill development in communication, coping, and conflict resolution, among others? Should we also teach a curriculum with greater emphasis on teamwork instead of competition since healthcare professionals interact with others in so many important ways?

Perhaps educators should congratulate improvements and consistency instead of reserving their praise for 'high achievers'. The key point is that once students understand the inherent occupational hazards, the impact of their personality, and the inevitable challenges they will face, perhaps they would develop greater self-awareness and be better prepared for the exciting yet challenging career to come.

This is an opportunity for future research, to see objectively what effect curriculum adjustments could have on burnout. By providing education on the risk factors contributing to burnout and other mental health problems before they arise, students might be prepared to seek help early when needed and develop their resilience.

> **ONCE STUDENTS UNDERSTAND THE INHERENT OCCUPATIONAL HAZARDS, THE IMPACT OF THEIR PERSONALITY, AND THE INEVITABLE CHALLENGES THEY WILL FACE, PERHAPS THEY WOULD DEVELOP GREATER SELF-AWARENESS AND BE BETTER PREPARED FOR THE EXCITING YET CHALLENGING CAREER TO COME.**

Locus of Control and Adaptability

A small hurdle for one person can present as a larger hurdle for someone else. This is particularly true for someone who may not have experienced certain adversities in life where they needed to develop their resilience. They may have never had to resort to an alternate plan 'B' or 'C' when the life path centered around plan 'A' failed. This person would be unaware of the necessity of resilience. A subtle change presenting as moral distress can build its effect over time. With the accumulation of distress, it can easily be seen how moral stressors incurred as a student, and never addressed, can become insurmountable as a physician in the first few years or middle of practice.

If the skills of resilience are never developed, then they cannot be readily accessed when needed. A societal norm tells us that if you work hard then predictable positive outcomes will ensue. Students attribute an outcome as completely within their control, with a markedly internal locus of control. The idea is that whatever amount of effort they put into a task, for example studying, they will achieve the direct and reflecting outcome [157]. Healthcare can be an extremely volatile environment, where outcomes are influenced by external factors, and at times in unpredictable ways. This can be seen particularly in acute settings such as the emergency department and inpatient hospital wards; physicians working in these locations are trained in specialties showing high rates of burnout. My prediction is that when someone is well attuned to having an internal locus of control, they must quickly become flexible in their locus of control, or they will struggle with outcomes occurring in a complex or chaotic type of environment. Perhaps the greatest illustration of the variable healthcare environment is the Cynefin framework, as seen below from The Canadian Society of Physician Leaders, and originally modified from an article in the Harvard Business Review [158]. In this article, Van Aerde and Gautam discuss the need for agile physician leadership when the healthcare environment changes to a chaotic environment, such as during the COVID-19 pandemic [159]. An understanding of the healthcare environment is also important when considering the locus of control. The environment is impacted by disorder, as indicated in the middle of the image below. This disorder can take a simple system to a complicated system, a complex system, and even chaotic system, in any order. In a simple system, there is a high level of agreement on best practices and actions are decided in a realm where the outcome, otherwise cause-and-effect, is known. When the system is complicated there is still a sense of order, but more experts are needed for its smooth operation, and there is usually more than one possible solution or outcome when deciding on the appropriate action to take. The complex system most closely depicts the environment of the healthcare system on a regular basis, where many complex elements interact with constant changes occurring. This consists of a space where there is less order and less agreement on the best course of action, mostly due to a lack of known cause-and-effect outcomes. In this environment there is constant ongoing learning and probing. In the adapted Cynefin framework this is labeled as emergent practice but described in a manner where there is still time to assess patterns or perform a small trial and make observations. The chaotic system consists of a crisis scenario where there is no time to probe possible outcomes, and the first step required is action rather than a plan. In chaotic systems, there are no patterns to observe, and the cause-and-effect of certain actions cannot be discerned. Such a system could be seen during the COVID-19 pandemic. In these forms of environments, it is hard to come to terms with the unknown if you have a strictly internal locus of control. In order to adapt, you need to be flexible, and willing to adjust your approach. There is a need for different leadership styles in each system. In the simple system where constraints are present in a fixed manner, there are protocols to follow and often there is one person in the position of control or command. An example of a simple system would be during resuscitation, which can often be practiced through simulation. In a complicated and complex system, the constraints are not as rigid as in a simple system, and the type of leadership that is needed is usually one of diverse collaboration, what the authors called distributive leadership. In chaotic systems, there are no constraints, and the situation requires quick action, often without time for collaborating or consulting others. Initially the form of leadership that works best is one of command, to establish control and order and attempt to move the system from chaotic into complex. To be successful in these environments you must be willing to adapt.

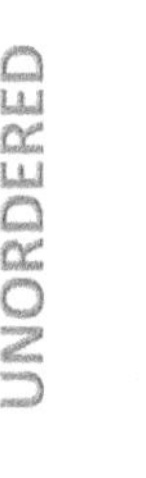

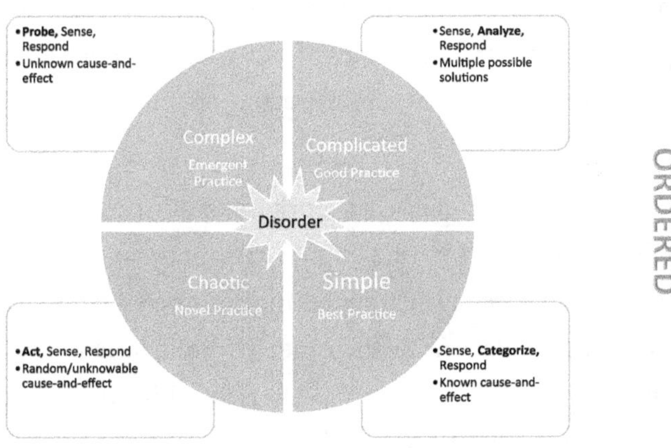

The Culture of Medicine and a Balance Between Positive or Negative Potentials

Physicians are incredibly dedicated and are drawn to serve others; this requires sacrifice which in turn must be carefully weighed or it can lead to them feeling deprived or taken advantage of [160].

The sacrifice is emotional, too. Physicians display compassion to patients and families while often suppressing their own emotions when processing difficult medical situations and outcomes. Such circumstances can feel so uniquely and personally isolating that over time, it contributes to emotional burnout (See image). Physicians sometimes experience intense suffering, called second victim syndrome (SVS), defined in 2000 by Dr. Wu, who used the term to describe the psychological trauma experienced by a physician, nurse, pharmacist, or other patient caregiver. This psychological trauma results from a disheartening adverse patient outcome, whether inadvertent, expected or unexpected, or even due to medical error [161].

SVS has occurred in healthcare workers of all specialties, but emergency medicine seems to have a higher risk because they often deal with acute patients, frequent life threatening conditions, and often must move quickly from one patient to the other without time for processing each event in between interactions [162]. After the shift, the events of the shift may weigh severely on the mind, like a tidal wave of emotions. Other health care personnel including nurses and pharmacists, deeply caring for patients, are far from immune to this syndrome [163]. The distress from SVS can contribute to burnout.

Certain components of medicine, that in and of themselves may not be seen as negative, could still be significant contributors to burnout [164].

The image below shows how a very positive value can potentially lead to burnout.

In an article by Dr. Nedrow and colleagues, they discussed that the desire to achieve excellence can result in perfectionism and a zero tolerance of mistakes; they termed this negative potential as *invincibility* [165].

Trainees can often succumb to something called imposter syndrome,

where despite good evaluations they battle recurring doubts in their own competence. A trainee might overcompensate to combat those doubts (omnipotence) [166].

The health care field can be particularly isolating because we focus on others with empathy and compassion, often without acknowledging our own feelings. Each of the four points seen in this image require an important balance so that the positive value does not turn into its negative potential. Our trainees and professional personnel need an acute awareness of these negative potentials, as well as effective ways to combat these possible transformations, which lead to burnout.

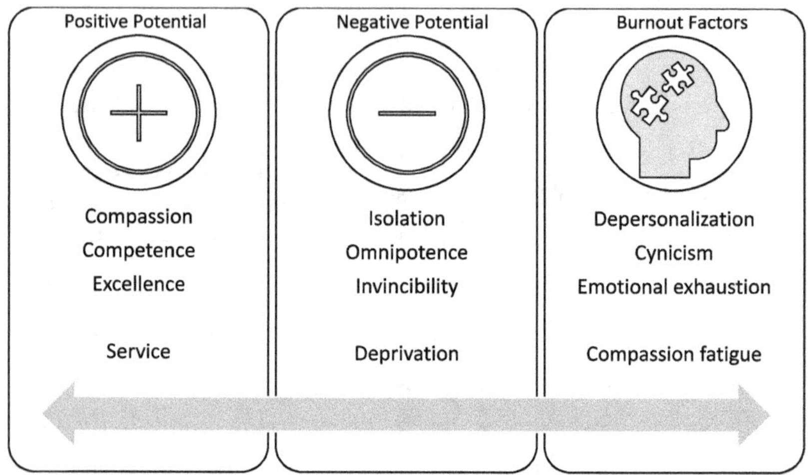

Key Chapter Points

- Provide education on the risk factors contributing to burnout and other mental health problems before they arise.
- Ensure anonymous access to mental health personnel is available.
- Discuss the components of the Resilience Framework practically.
- Training should include education on personality traits, hazards of the work environment, communication, coping, and conflict resolution.
- Understand the impact of disorder within the healthcare environment and on potential outcomes. Successfully adapt your approach and decision-making style.
- Incorporate education on negative potentials within the culture of medicine, SVS, and imposter syndrome. Include skills training with effective and practical tools to combat this possible transformation for healthcare personnel.

Discover your personality traits

CHAPTER 10:
INTERVENTIONS AND COPING METHODS

"As a student, I started to experience imposter syndrome. I sought help from a mentor and realized that I wasn't alone in what I was going through."

Goals: Educate on coping mechanisms while promoting and utilizing evidence-based interventions to reduce burnout.

In general, you could predict that burnout would be associated with poor stress coping mechanisms such as increased drug and alcohol use and increased suicidal ideation and suicide attempts (I want to be clear that burnout is distinct from stress, and distinct from job dissatisfaction). Actually, when comparing physicians to the general population, they do not tend to turn to drug and alcohol abuse more when stressed and burned out, but they were found to have a higher use of prescription drugs and self-medicating [167]. In a survey of health professionals including nurses, dentists, pharmacists, and physicians, their level of alcohol use was not greater than the general population [168].

In 1976, a psychologist and researcher, Christina Maslach, began researching the concept of burnout while interviewing service workers, (people in occupations helping others) including health care, social services, mental health, criminal justice, and education [169]. The Maslach Burnout Inventory (MBI) was developed out of her research and is a widely accepted tool worldwide to investigate burnout through research, individual self-assessment, or group comparisons although it is not diagnostic [170]. The MBI looks at the three results of burnout: emotional exhaustion, depersonalization, and decreased personal accomplishment. Other burnout questionnaires measure burnout: some measure only one aspect such as exhaustion, some differentiate exhaustion into physical and emotional, and other measures have added dimensions like fatigue, guilt, or interpersonal strain [171].

Burnout, stress, and depression. Are they synonymous?

Burnout syndrome goes far beyond stress alone as each individual's response and tolerance varies (resulting in stress); it involves exhaustion, a decreased sense of personal accomplishment, and sometimes a withdrawing into de-personal interactions with others in the workplace [172].

Some believe that burnout may simply be depression; however, studies show that burnout is distinct from depression, though the two are related and can co-exist [173].

Often, when someone attempts suicide, the discussion is lead to a discussion of depression. Suicidal thoughts, called ideation, is only one diagnostic criterion to determine depression, and depression is only one psychiatric diagnosis ascribed to the presence of suicidal thoughts. The absence of depression does not mean there is not a risk of suicidal ideation. Other psychological illnesses can result in it as well: anxiety disorders, bipolar disorder, substance use disorder, and various personality disorders [174]. Combinations of more than one of these issues, such as substance use disorder plus a personality disorder, can increase the risk.

Family or friends of healthcare clinicians who committed suicide often had no idea the person was experiencing mental stressors, or that they were 'depressed' to such an extent [175]. You might think that physicians are better able to hide their psychological stress because they understand depression professionally. That is not the case. If health professionals can hide it, then depression is a diagnosis based on symptoms that can be suppressed at will. It is more likely that physicians and health professionals are in a state of denial or avoidance and that the signs of depression or distress have been missed and not hidden [176]. Even physicians are sometimes unable to recognize depression in colleagues [177].

Common signs of possible psychological distress, that when seen should warrant further discussion, can be found in the table below. [178]

Signs of Acute Suicide Risk	Additional Warning Signs
Threatening to hurt or kill him or herself, or talking of wanting to hurt or kill him/herself; and or,	Increased substance (alcohol or drug) use
Looking for ways to kill him/herself by seeking access to firearms, available pills, or other means; and/or,	No reason for living; no sense of purpose in life
Talking or writing about death, dying or suicide, when these actions are out of the ordinary.	Anxiety, agitation, unable to sleep or sleeping all of the time
	Feeling trapped – like there's no way out
	Hopelessness
	Withdrawal from friends, family, and society
	Rage, uncontrolled anger, seeking revenge
	Acting reckless or engaging in risky activities, seemingly without thinking
	Dramatic mood changes
	Giving away prized possessions or seeking long-term care for pets

Dealing with Critical, Dying Patients

Dealing with death and dying patients can certainly add to stress and burnout in health care professionals. A study of 1,156 physicians showed that physicians who were burned out, felt emotionally exhausted when dealing with dying patients [179]. The study wasn't clear whether the physician's emotional exhaustion came as a result of overall burnout, or if their struggle to cope with dying patients contributed to burnout. Likely, it is a combination of both. Interestingly, physicians who worked in end-of-life specialties did not have higher rates of burnout than those in other specialties. Thus, a career path that has people working directly with dying patients does not equate to a higher rate of burnout. Individual religious beliefs and coping mechanisms do however make a difference [180].

Coping Mechanisms

A common classification system, identifies coping strategies as either emotion-focused or problem-focused [181]. The problem-focused strategy is to develop a plan. "How will I solve the problem? What options and actions could potentially help?" In an emotion-focused approach, the aim is to decrease your emotional response to the stressor. That might mean distancing, self-isolation, wishful thinking, denial, acceptance, rethinking the situation, seeking emotional support, or turning to religion [182].

People can respond to the same stressor either way, depending on whether they believe that the stressor must be endured or if something constructive can be done to deal with it. Individuals may tend to use one approach versus the other [183].

Does the type of coping strategies you choose affect the level or risk of burnout? Absolutely. Avoidance is one coping technique that is particularly problematic and associated with stress [184]. In fact, some emotion-focused coping correlates directly with higher burnout in all of its manifestations [185]. This wasn't true of all emotion-focused coping strategies however, seeking support, acceptance, reappraisal, and religion had no bearing on increasing burnout. Seeking support certainly helps a person stay connected to colleagues and others (as did religion) and thus depersonalization and feelings of reduced personal accomplishment were low. People who cope through reappraisal had low emotional exhaustion and low reduced personal accomplishment. [186].

I would recommend that you add a few different coping techniques to your arsenal. Do not avoid problems, but when the emotional tension increases, it is time to exhaust all avenues available to you, in order to find relief, like seeking support from others, or turning to religion, to allow you to see your problems and the world from a broader perspective. Seeking help from others can provide you with valuable insight, new perspectives, and support from those who care about you. Don't give up when someone may not offer the support you need, but reach out to other people, as each person is different, some may be better able to assist or support you than others. Discussing problems with others can also allow you to reappraise the situation from multiple angles. Overall, you should try to develop a plan to overcome the problem.

Insight into Burnout Interventions

Increasingly popular in recent years are techniques called mindfulness-based interventions, which includes mindfulness-based stress reduction (MBSR), mindfulness-based cognitive therapy (MBCT), dialectal behavior therapy (DBT), and acceptance and commitment therapy

(ACT) [187]. Mindfulness-based interventions are derived from the application of Buddhist meditation and philosophy [188].

The goal of mindfulness-based interventions is twofold: to resolve habits that lead to damaging emotions and increase positive ones [189]. The earliest mindfulness-based intervention, known as MBSR, was developed in 1979 – integrating Buddhist practices to reduce stress by increasing awareness. Some studies have also found it helpful to reduce anxiety and depression [190]. Outcomes have varied on the effect of MBSR to reduce burnout in healthcare providers, although it has been found to reduce stress, anxiety, and depression [191]. Further research is necessary in this specific area.

Targeted interventions for burnout that are directed at the organizational level rather than at the individual, lead to a greater reduction in overall burnout and have a longer lasting, positive effect [192]. The study by Panagioti and colleagues, looked at results from multiple studies researching burnout interventions, termed a meta-analysis. They saw that individual interventions supported or provided at the organizational level also had longer lasting outcomes to reduce burnout. Individual interventions included mindfulness-based stress reduction techniques, and education on self-confidence and communication skills. Interventions at the organizational level included modifications and reduction to workload, enhanced teamwork, and leadership through discussion meetings [193].

TARGETED INTERVENTIONS FOR BURNOUT THAT ARE DIRECTED AT THE ORGANIZATIONAL LEVEL RATHER THAN AT THE INDIVIDUAL, LEAD TO A GREATER REDUCTION IN OVERALL BURNOUT AND HAVE A LONGER LASTING, POSITIVE EFFECT.

Organizational interventions are also more effective than individual measures in reducing overall burnout [194]. Both organizational and individual interventions were able to reduce burnout domains such as emotional exhaustion or depersonalization. Further research is needed to learn which interventions are more effective in reducing burnout than others.

Professional coaching intervention was randomly tried for 88 physicians and resulted in a significant decrease in overall burnout and emotional exhaustion, improved their quality of life and resilience. The physicians had 3.5 hours of professional coaching over 5 months [195]. The authors pointed out that coaching does not replace the need for organizational interventions, nor did their study determine how long these improvements in burnout remained.

Key Chapter Points

- Burnout and stress can lead to poor coping mechanisms. However, burnout has been shown to be distinct from stress and from a lack of job satisfaction.
- The Maslach Burnout Inventory (MBI) is a widely accepted tool worldwide to investigate burnout.
- The MBI looks at the 3 aspects of burnout – emotional exhaustion, depersonalization, and decreased personal accomplishment.
- It seems that inherently dealing with death and dying patients does not equate to a higher rate of burnout.
- Both individual and organizational interventions have shown to decrease burnout domains. In comparison, organizational interventions might lead to greater reduction in overall burnout.

- Research is needed on interventions to reduce burnout and their duration of effect.

Learn More

CHAPTER 11:
DEBT AND FINANCIAL BURDENS

"It's simple supply and demand: medical schools demand tuition at a maximized cost, knowing lenders will provide loans to a surplus of students who are willing to pay."

Goals: Consider the impact of the financial burden on students as it relates to burnout and abandoning the professional pursuit; utilize all avenues to integrate medical graduates into the healthcare system and reduce shortages.

The education costs of medical training are uniquely sky high; the pressure of those costs in and of themselves are huge contributors to burnout [196]. The burden of debt surmounted to an average of $190, 000 per medical student in 2017, and can sometimes be greater than $250, 000 [197].

Some graduates change their career and specialty choice over the issue of debt. Those with larger debts may move away from careers with a lower income, such as primary care [198]. That should get our attention, considering the increasing demand for greater numbers of physicians in primary care. The Association of American Medical Colleges (AAMC) predicted that in the US, 43,100 primary care positions and 61,800 non-primary care positions will be needed by 2030 [199]. Canada has experienced a decrease in the inflow of over 5,000 physicians from 1994 to 2000, most likely due to a series of restrictions and policies that eliminated the rotating internship program in 1993 and increased the length of training requirements [200]. Decreased intake of International Medical Graduates (IMGs), increased retirements, a 10 percent reduction in the number of medical school positions, and migration of some physicians to the US have all contributed to the shortage [201].

It is obvious that the educational bodies have not done enough to resolve these shortages. In fact, the changes made to the training system over the years have propagated what is now labeled a shortage. But what do they mean by shortage? It is important to understand where the bottleneck is occurring.

Surplus of New Physicians, Shortage of Training Positions

Each year, thousands of new doctors are left stranded after medical school graduation when not matched into a residency training position. In 2021 there were 9,155 doctors in the US that went unmatched. That included over 3,000 doctors from US medical schools and over 5,500 US citizens [202]. Some of this may be due to high competition; however, there is also a clear lack of training positions to accommodate the number of physicians that are needed. There were 35,194 first year positions in the US in 2021, almost a thousand more than in 2020. At the same time, the number of applicants increased by almost 4,000 from 2020 to 2021. The number of residency positions has only marginally increased each year while the number of applicants is rising at a much faster pace.

At this time, these highly knowledgeable new medical doctors have no interim options that would allow them to contribute to the medical workforce. This means that nearly 20 percent of newly invested doctors must scramble their way through a year or more of uncertainty with odd jobs or research work. They are unable to engage in patient care or further clinical training due to legislation. If unmatched to a program the following year, they may be in 'limbo' for multiple years, at which time the competition grows again as more new doctors apply for the same positions.

This also occurs in Canada, though on a smaller but equally significant scale, as there are fewer medical schools and fewer residency training positions than in the US. In Canada, there were 3,365 residency positions in 2021, which was 32 positions less than the number offered in 2020; the number of applicants totaled 4,834 and 25 percent of those who submitted a rank list went unmatched [203] [204]. In 2020, there were nearly 400 fewer applicants yet 25 percent still went unmatched [205].

The shortage of training positions does not account for the number of students that are in medical training who have trained in medicine abroad and returned as International Medical Graduates. When the number of medical schools within the United States or Canada reaches capacity, students may resort to applying for schools overseas to complete their medical education. Returning to the US or Canada is complicated by the lack of training positions. Their exam scores, competence and patient outcomes are on par with North American graduates, but they struggle to match with training programs as well [206].

The shortage of physicians – while truly occurring due to early retirements and burnout – does not mean that there is a shortage of medical students to train as physicians. This false pretense is used as a basis to hire and train larger amounts of 'advanced practice' specialist nurses, physician assistants etc. to fill the supposed physician shortage. I believe that if there were an increase in residency training positions, there would likely be enough competent physicians for the positions in shortage.

This raises the question, *what about the underserved rural areas that may seem difficult to recruit staff to?* In this case, let's incentivize movement to those locations. The government can accept those who are willing to work in the underserved areas and provide financial incentives, loan forgiveness, or sponsored visa opportunities for these positions, because the truth of the matter is that physicians who trained abroad are often willing to work in rural locations when emigrating from around the World or as near as neighboring Canada, in the case of the US. Legislative bodies can provide return for service contracts after residency training to motivate these physicians to stay.

The current healthcare system is not structured to reduce physician shortages in North America. Rather, we lose so much potential as new doctors, year after year, are unable to find residency training. Unmatched new doctors who could be assisting and seeing patients under supervision, and keeping their clinical skills sharp, can't obtain any form of licensure which would allow them to do so! If unmatched to a residency program, this potential workforce goes untapped. Nurse practitioners on the other hand, can obtain an independent license in over 23 states, but they will have completed less clinical training hours than that of medical school graduates, who are new doctors, unable to obtain a license without a residency training program [207]. This reality is depicted in the image below. Without opportunities to maintain their clinical skills until the following year's residency match, the cycle continues. It's easy to see that if this continues into consecutive years, many physicians are forced into non-clinical career positions or

THE SHORTAGE OF PHYSICIANS – WHILE TRULY OCCURRING DUE TO EARLY RETIREMENTS AND BURNOUT – DOES NOT MEAN THAT THERE IS A SHORTAGE OF MEDICAL STUDENTS TO TRAIN AS PHYSICIANS.

completely change their career path altogether after 8+ years of education.

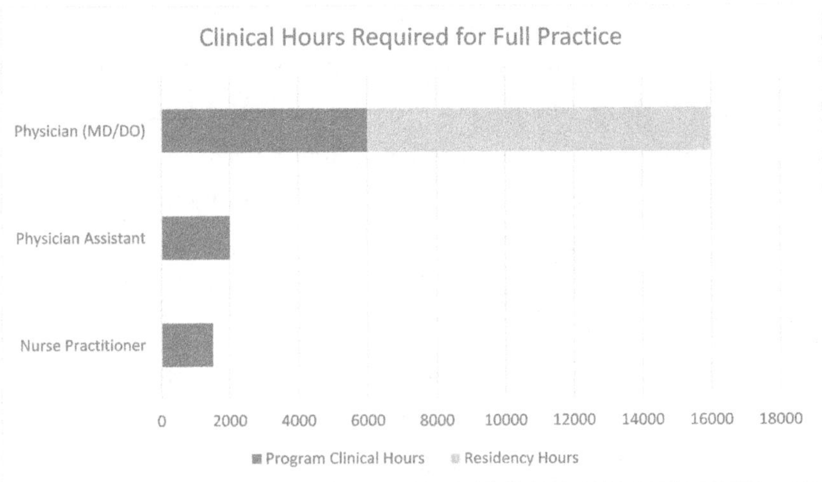

This issue has largely been overlooked, and only as of 2014 has the state of Missouri developed an assistant physician license (allowing new graduates/doctors more opportunities to serve in the shorted workforce, especially in underserved areas) [208]. There are at least three other states which have developed a similar license, each with differing restrictions/qualifications. There should be immediate widespread reform to curb this 'shortage' and integrate competent medical graduates into the healthcare workforce.

You can see how all of these factors can quite easily contribute to burnout. New doctors are strained with insurmountable debt when they graduate medical school. They must then navigate into a residency position fraught with logistical challenges. They are influenced to choose a career that will provide enough income to decrease this debt, and if they go unmatched into residency, this adds to psychological stressors and societal untapped resources. All of this occurs while at the other end of the spectrum practicing physicians are being forced from their jobs due burnout, which leads to a shortage of doctors. However, a short-sighted solution is to train and hire staff who require less training and carry less costs to replace them, when in fact there are medical graduates searching for clinical opportunities, who can competently perform many tasks to relieve the health system burden. Thus, this misleading information depicting only one aspect of the physician shortage is propagated. This also triggers many students to eagerly apply to medical schools assuming ease in the process of securing a job, while the number of residency training positions do not reflect this student increase. The gap between the large number of medical graduates and available residency positions will continue to widen and the cycle continues.

Key Chapter Points

- The financial debt burden can often be greater than $250, 000 which strongly correlates with increased burnout.
- Increase the number of residency training positions to account for the surplus of medical students.
- Integrate the 8,000+ new doctors who go without residency placements each year into the US and Canadian healthcare systems.

SECTION 4:

Consequences of Burnout for the Individual

I f we want to know why burnout is such a pressing issue, we need to look no further than the far-reaching consequences it has. Individual consequences are numerous. The ones I will touch upon in this section include physical and mental illness, such as the deadliness of fatigue. Increased suicide risk, injuries, medical errors, and attrition. All of these consequences not only impact individuals, but also patients and the health care organizations.

CHAPTER 12:
MEDICAL ERRORS

"Even I could've become a doctor."

Goals: Shed light on the effect of burnout on one's increased perception of medical errors.

Some studies show that the quality of patient care becomes affected when staff members are burned out [209]. Although it is difficult to objectively monitor medical errors by individuals, equally troubling is that those who identify as being burned out have the *perception* that they are making more errors [210]. If you weren't convinced, this is the reason this book and this topic are so important!

Studies do show that burnout correlates with errors, although the extent to which the severity of burnout affects errors has yet to be objectively determined [211]. There is believed to be a cyclical relationship between medical errors and burnout [212]. If medical errors increase, it may cause burnout, and vice versa; when burnout increases, this could lead to increased medical errors. Many of the studies looking at error and burnout rely on self-reporting by the professionals, so it can be tough to make objective or empirical conclusions. However, one study of 1145 physicians in a US academic medical center found that physician depersonalization was the primary cause of increases in patient complaints, not emotional exhaustion, or overall burnout [213]. Interestingly, emotional exhaustion was often noted by physicians at the same time patients were noting increased satisfaction with the communication levels of their primary care physician. This may be due to physicians, who provide more time and care to patients, becoming emotionally exhausted.

A meta-analysis study looked at the results of 82 studies from various healthcare providers and found that emotional exhaustion had a strong relationship with the quality of patient care [214]. Burned out providers were perceived by patients to provide a lower quality of care.

It is quite possible that burnout among nurses might be a better predictor of how patients would rate quality of care, since nurses typically have more face time with patients than other healthcare professionals [215]. One study of nurses in 540 nursing homes in the US, found that those who were suffering from emotional exhaustion (~30 percent), reported an inability to perform necessary care due to time or resource constraints, at a rate of five times more often than those who were not emotionally exhausted [216]. Time and resource constraints are burnout drivers, as discussed in section 2, chapter 4. There are limitations to any study, as many of them look at a cross-section of population over time (and certainly there are other factors that influence quality of care), but there is a basis on these general conclusions about exhaustion, burnout, and care.

Litigation or dismissal are common consequences of medical error, but unless caused by a deliberate error or negligence, these responses fail to prevent the same errors from happening again. Patient safety is a complex issue. Often the prevalence of errors indicates that there is a larger system error that is responsible [217].

Errors can be described as active or latent failures [218]. Plane crashes, for example, could result from an active error, such as a pilot's mistake. A latent error would be outside the pilot's control, such a design flaw, lack of maintenance, etc.

In healthcare, active errors can include breaches in safety defenses, unsafe actions by the person in direct contact with a patient (e.g., nurse, physician, nursing attendant, technician, etc.). However, latent issues contributing to an employee's error might include poor organizational structure, scheduling issues, or lack of training.

Latent errors often have delayed consequences and can frequently go unrecognized, leading to many individual active failures from employees who make mistakes while put into a flawed system that hasn't been fixed. Latent errors and conditions can come to pass so gradually that employees adapt to them and then become blind to them – seeing them as normal [219]. Latent organizational issues can make the system error prone, and lead to repeated active errors [220]. This is why, in cases when considering any error or adverse event, it is so important to have an objective investigation of both the incident and potential root causes.

Hindsight Bias and Medical Errors

"If I were in your shoes ...!"

Whether you are a clinician or an athlete, miss a diagnosis or miss a shot on goal – there will always be that someone who will state your incompetence or point out how they could have done it better. This chapter begins with the quote 'Even I could've become a doctor,' made by an administrator after a clinician error. I know that the administrator didn't really share the desire to become a doctor. The disturbing underlying premise of the statement is clear: *if physicians can make mistakes, then they aren't really doctors.*

What people don't see, is the history of the clinician's excellence, the years of health restored, or statistics that would serve to demonstrate how often a clinician got the diagnoses correct. Back to sports, fans watched basketball legend Michael Jordan perform with Hall of Fame credentials. He said that he was entrusted with the last second shot 26 times in his career and missed! If that's all you saw, then you wouldn't be aware of all those he made prior. You would not know how much work was put in, or how many years of training was undertaken to get to that point in his career.

The moment something does not go right, onlookers typically have something negative to say. Following my personal experiences, I think it's probably best to anticipate the negativity and be appreciative of sympathy or empathy than be surprised by negativity. Being aware of this human tendency towards criticism can help us avoid shock or surprise when it comes; that doesn't mean we need to focus in on the negative or let it negatively affect our perspective.

WHETHER YOU ARE A CLINICIAN OR AN ATHLETE, MISS A DIAGNOSIS OR MISS A SHOT ON GOAL – THERE WILL ALWAYS BE THAT SOMEONE WHO WILL STATE YOUR INCOMPETENCE OR POINT OUT HOW THEY COULD HAVE DONE IT BETTER.

Hindsight bias is the name given by psychologists to "the tendency, after an event has occurred, to overestimate the extent to which the outcome could have been foreseen" [221]. This kind of bias represents a commonplace, human reflex, which I have termed the *demise-reflex*. We've all been guilty of it, making a negative statement almost automatically when someone makes an error. What is a reflex? Just like when a physician taps the tendon of your kneecap and your leg jumps, the demise-reflex works similarly. Maybe you're watching your favorite sport and the athlete misses a pass or a shot on goal, and your reaction is that 'he/she should have done this instead', or 'if I were there, I could have made that play'. This aspect of human nature has far-reaching implications beyond that of sports or events from which we are far removed.

How can we increase awareness and learn to shut off this reflex towards others, particularly within healthcare? We must consciously remind ourselves that errors occur as a result of multiple factors. There are external and situational factors as well as internal and individual factors at play in any given scenario. People do not purposely set out to make an error, especially one that impacts another person. We are all human beings and therefore prone to human error – nobody is immune from this inherent condition. Even with immense practice and repetition, perfection is subjective, depending on whose standard you compare to. Mistakes are therefore inevitable, particularly when external or situational forces are out of control.

We can only perfect what is within our control, but since no one lives within a vacuum, unexpected things can and do happen.

When at the receiving end of the demise-reflex, what approach should you take? If you submit emotionally to the criticism as stated, you'll add fuel to the fires of self-doubt, low self-esteem, or depression that assault your every thought and decision.

In the resiliency framework I presented earlier in the book, you can add another set of questions to ask yourself to help respond to the 'demise-reflex.'

1. Was the error I made done so with a malicious intent?
2. Have I changed a key approach or habit that used to produce positive outcomes?
3. What can I learn from this error or situation?

In this way, not only do you hold yourself accountable, but you also don't have to take on the negative accountability from others. In sports, referees can check their performance against video reviews. If we make an error personally in healthcare roles, we can gain insight from external sources such as the patient or family.

Using the questions will help you frame your response or reaction to the opinions of others. The first two questions that we ask ourselves are self-explanatory. If an error was made consciously with a malicious intent, then you need to seek some professional input for a deeper, possibly psychological, issue that needs to be addressed. The second question identifies whether you changed something that had been working well.

I purposely did not write a question regarding or assessing the level of effort, because as stated in the previous chapter, many people have the mentality that every outcome is a result of their personal effort, maintaining an internal locus of control. In other words, if they were to ask themselves in hindsight whether they gave their best effort, the very fact that there was a negative result would mean to them that they must have given a substandard or low effort. They would automatically answer the question of whether they gave their best effort with a 'no' since it did not achieve a positive result. For this reason, I don't think it will be constructive to ask ourselves whether we gave our best. Rather, it's better to focus on our approach or habits, and then we can take actions to make corrections or promote improvement.

A review of each error situation is important in helping foster the necessary change. Recommendations might include making adjustments to increase sleep or cultivating a system of checks and balances. After this analysis and necessary change(s) has been identified, the next question we should ask ourselves when a mistake occurs is, 'what can we learn from this error or situation?'

What we can learn from an error involves not only how we might prevent it from occurring again, but also what we learned about ourselves in the process. You gain insight on how you react emotionally when you realize that an error has occurred: "Did I get angry, sad, move into denial, or another emotional response?" Can you accept the notion that as a human being you are fallible? Introspection is key to our mental well-being; by acknowledging our emotions we can be better prepared to address them, handle potential mistakes in the future, and overall increase our resiliency.

Key Chapter Points

- Those who have identified as being burnt out often report an increased prevalence of errors and an increased perception of making errors.
- Human beings are fallible. When errors occur take an introspective look and acknowledge your feelings.
- Questions to ask ourselves, and aid our response, when we are on the receiving end of the demise-reflex and hindsight bias:
  - Was the error I made done so with a malicious intent?
  - Have I changed a key approach or habit that used to produce positive outcomes?
  - What can I learn from this error or situation?

CHAPTER 13:
EXHAUSTION

*"At times, I'm jealous of that patient
sedated on the operating table."*

Goals: Understand the impact of increased insomnia and fatigue on individuals.

There are laws in place to protect certain high-stakes professionals such as airline pilots and aircrew members against being overworked or over-stressed. According to the Federal Aviation Administration (FAA), airline pilots are required to have ten hours of rest between shifts with a mandatory eight hours consecutive for sleep [222]. Pilots also require annual fatigue-related education and training, and every two years, this training must be updated. The airline carrier and the pilot work in a joint effort to prevent fatigue in order to protect the public. The airline carrier is responsible, organizationally, to provide an environment in which time for sufficient recovery periods is allowed and encouraged. The FAA even added restrictions on flight duty when crew members' internal clocks were likely at their low rhythm, which usually occurs at night [223]. During this low circadian rhythm, they found that flight crew members experienced lower performance. When longer duty hours are needed, the airline carrier is then responsible to provide staff adequate rest facilities and additional crew members to ensure an alert staff member provides coverage. Crew members working at night are required to have at least a 2-hour rest period per night, when working consecutive night shifts (a maximum of 5 nights) – concluding that performance was significantly affected without it.

Why am I telling you all of this? We all understand the need for pilots to be fully awake, rested, and alert. But here's the thing, there are no such universal rules, regulations, or mandatory fatigue education within healthcare!

Clinicians are not immune to the effects of fatigue, and human lives are very much at stake. Why couldn't similar fatigue education be provided to address its effects and provide countermeasures for those in our profession? Regulations regarding work hours are important, as the FAA has demonstrated, even critical when so many people's lives are at stake.

What about clinicians? Why are there so few regulations regarding healthcare professional work hours? A surgeon or cardiovascular specialist's responsibilities require fine motor movements while attempting to save someone's life; perhaps the patient is suffering from a gunshot wound or heart attack. I'm quite sure that if the FAA were in charge of healthcare, they would safeguard those physicians with fatigue training and other measures for the good of the industry and the patients we care for. Within healthcare, there is so much more to be done in terms of better technology, education, and overall effort to reduce the fatigue that can decrease performance and risk many lives.

The Effect of Sleep Loss on Functional Ability

Chronic sleep loss can cause a person to unintentionally fall asleep during the day, a syndrome called sleep propensity. What's surprising is that it doesn't actually take much sleep loss for this to happen.

One study restricted healthy individuals to a limit of 4, 6, or 8 hours of sleep for 14 consecutive nights. Another group was restricted to 3 full nights without any sleep. The two groups were studied and compared. The first group performed poorly on a test (Psychomotor Vigilance Task (PVT) test) of behavior, motor alertness, and memory, and the less sleep they received, the worse their scores. [224]. Those who were restricted to either 6 or 4 hours of sleep for 14 days showed significant lapses in their alertness and working memory, the same as those who did not sleep at all for 1 or 2 days respectively.

They also tested ability to complete a serial addition and subtraction task, and the 4-hour group after 14 days performed the same as if they had gone a full day without sleeping. This impairment was consistent throughout the day, as opposed to just certain times of the day. It was found that in each of the 4 groups, being awake for over a mean time of ~15.8 hours resulted in significant lapses in their performance [225]. ~8.2 hours of sleep was needed to prevent this lapse.

When the participants in the 4 hour and 6-hour group were asked to indicate their subjective level of sleepiness, their responses of 'slight sleepiness' were similar, although their performance measures worsened the less sleep they received. This indicates a possible lack of insight as to their functionality.

> **BEING AWAKE FOR OVER A MEAN TIME OF ~15.8 HOURS RESULTED IN SIGNIFICANT LAPSES IN THEIR PERFORMANCE. ~8.2 HOURS OF SLEEP WAS NEEDED TO PREVENT THIS LAPSE.**

Another study [226] found similar results. This experiment restricted groups to 3, 5, 7, or 9 hours in bed for 7 days, and then allowed each group 3 days of 8 hours *sleep recovery*. Healthcare organizations and professionals should be gravely concerned by these findings, because sleep recovery did not happen! Those who were in the 7-hour and 5-hour restriction groups demonstrated no improvement in impairment for the 3 days of 8 hours of sleep. The group restricted to 3-hours of sleep for 7 days demonstrated improvements in performance that stabilized at a level similar to those who only had 5 or 7 hours of sleep. Volunteers in the 9 hours' sleep group had performance levels that remained constant throughout the experiment [227].

In Australia, researchers compared the performance levels from sleep deprivation to that of alcohol consumption [228]. They found that performance level test results on volunteers who were awake for between 17 to 19 hours was equivalent to that of individuals who consumed alcohol resulting in a blood alcohol level of 0.05 percent. Decreasing sleep amounts further resulted in performance levels matching those with 0.1 percent blood alcohol concentration. That decreased performance showed up in tests of accuracy, reaction speed, and hand-eye coordination, among others.

A similar study that compared sleep deprivation and blood alcohol levels indicated performance impairment after sleep deprivation, equivalent to 0.05 percent blood alcohol level. They concluded that people are at high risk if they drive after 20 hours without sleep [229]. The chart below demonstrates a person's risk of car accident after obtaining certain amounts of sleep. The car crash risk more than doubles if sleep is reduced from 5-6 hours to between 4-5 hours of sleep [230]. Deeply concerning for our profession is that the risk of car crashes, when sleeping less than 4 hours, is 11 times greater than those who obtain more than 7 hours of sleep!

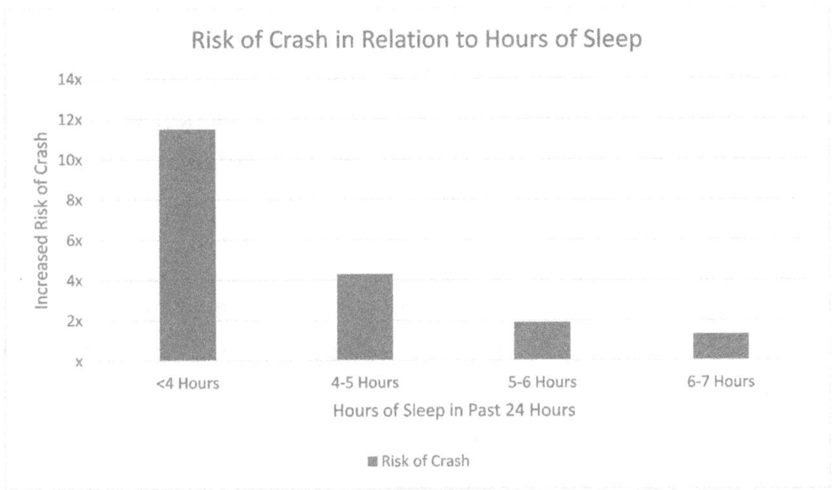

A survey of over 2,700 first year residents physicians (interns) found that after working an extended shift (over 24 hours) they had double the odds of being in a car crash and reached 5 times the number of near-miss accidents, as opposed to when working a non-extended shift [231]. Each time an extended shift was scheduled, it increased the rate of vehicle crashes by approximately 9 percent per month. Interns also reported falling asleep while driving or while stopped, although it should be noted that microsleeps can typically go unnoticed by the person.

You can see how fatigue from sleep deprivation is a grave concern, particularly within healthcare where this is so common.

Resident physicians on extended overnight shifts had significantly less sleep, low performance, and alertness between those working night shifts than those on day shifts [232]. When on-call, interns slept for an average of only 2.1 hours, and 17.5 percent of the time – *they didn't sleep at all*. When scheduled for an overnight call, residents were typically on shift for 30 hours. Interns on day shifts, by contrast, slept 6.9 hours in the evenings. Not surprisingly, residents demonstrated decreased alertness on PVT testing the following morning after on-call shifts, particularly within the first hour after waking. In fact, the level of alertness in those who slept and were tested within the first hour of waking was not much different than residents who did not sleep at all! This hour time frame of reduced performance is termed 'sleep inertia.'

Interns who were allowed to nap from midnight to 3 am or from 3 am to 6 am without their pager or cell phones (though the senior resident could awaken them when urgent) were much benefited, showing lower attention lapses on the PVT. These residents on average got 0.5 to 0.9 hours of more sleep than those who were not in the protected sleep group [233].

Our medical training needs to do better in directing and preparing trainees for their practice after graduation. Organizational skills, work life balance, and sleep hygiene deserve important emphasis on an individual and organizational level. Graduates will be expected to set their work schedule and balance life affairs after having little control over these issues while in training [234]. Leaders in healthcare and medical training must communicate the importance of sleep, recognizing burnout and depression, make necessary policy changes, and formulate strategies to combat fatigue and burnout within the healthcare system [235].

The Effects of Sleep Deprivation

Why is there so much more emphasis on fatigue prevention in aviation compared to healthcare? Of course, it is due to the very real immediate danger for masses of people. Hundreds of people's lives on the plane and on the ground are in jeopardy if the airplane were to crash.

Healthcare organizations, and the general public for that matter, may not view the high stakes issue of fatigue in our profession as a serious one. A fatigued physician risks the immediate life of the patient and impacts their family members and friends. Both the physician and all of their patients are affected. Without acknowledging the widespread hazards of fatigue, society is sacrificing our clinicians as more and more suffer from burnout or depression which has all kinds of consequences. Burnout, depression, and suicide affects us all. For example, a family physician treats multiple generations within a family, and on average that can include over 2,000 patients [236]. If that physician burns out from occupational pressures, these effects are felt by many people within a community beyond the immediate patients.

Key Chapter Points

- Education on the effects of fatigue should be provided within all healthcare personnel training.
- Shift hours should be structured to allow for adequate sleep. Fatigue from sleep deprivation leads to decrease performance, alertness, and can result in microsleeps.
- During on-call shifts sleeping time should be protected and routine interruptions discouraged.
- There is a balance between shift length, maintaining continuity of care, and minimizing errors. Continuous shift work without adequate breaks can contribute to burnout.

CHAPTER 14:
MENTAL (UN)WELLNESS

"I'm pretty sure I've been having runs of PVC's all day."

Goals: Understand how burnout increases the risk of physical and mental illnesses.

A 2019 NHS survey indicated that 40.3 percent of medical staff reported that work-related stress resulted in physical manifestations, such as generally feeling unwell; this was an increase from 36.8 percent in 2016 [237].

The consequences of burnout therefore affect not only patients, but lead to personal consequences for the staff themselves, such as increased risk for cardiovascular disease and other health concerns, and possibly decreased overall survival [238]. Consequences also include insomnia, use of drugs and alcohol, increased injuries at work, and suicide [239].

Statistics from studies vary, but one study of physicians with burnout showed an almost 200 percent greater chance of suicidal ideation [240]. Multiple studies have shown a relationship between burnout and much higher suicidal ideation – independent of depression – and find that suicidal thoughts subsided when burnout improved and that suicidal thoughts were less frequent in those without burnout

SUICIDAL IDEATION AND SUICIDE ITSELF, OCCUR AT A MUCH HIGHER RATE IN THE HEALTHCARE PROFESSION THAN THE GENERAL POPULATION.

[241]. However, another study surveying 1,354 physicians on levels of burnout and suicidal ideation, found that burnout was not the primary factor

associated with suicidal ideation in and of itself, after adjusting for symptoms of depression [242]. It may be that depression and not burnout is more to blame for suicidal ideation, although the relationship with burnout and depression requires further research. The primary point is this: suicidal ideation and suicide itself, occur at a much higher rate in the healthcare profession than the general population.

Suicide and Suicidal Thoughts

In Canadian physicians, 29 percent of physicians surveyed indicated high levels of burnout, and 32 percent screened positive for depression. Eight percent of the 2,547 surveyed admitted to suicidal ideation in the past year, and more were female physicians (9 percent versus 7 percent of males). Those in their first 5 years of practice reported the highest prevalence of suicidal ideation [243]. Suicidal ideation was also higher among residents. Fifteen percent of 400 resident physicians reported suicidal ideation in the past year and 27 percent in their lifetime.

In the US, 43.9 percent of physicians reported burnout, and 41.7 percent screened positive for depression. 6.5 percent of 5,445 physicians surveyed indicated that they had had thoughts of suicide in the past year [244]. There was a higher risk for physicians that were younger (median age 50), in practice for less time (median 17 years), and female (7.6 percent versus 5.9 percent for males). Looking at each group separately, 9.6 percent of physicians aged 25-34 indicated suicidal ideation, and 8.8 percent of physicians in practice for between 5 to less than 10 years, although not statistically significant.

A similar survey of 7,378 nurses found that 5.5 percent had suicidal ideation in the past year. Of the total that was surveyed, 38.2 percent reported burnout, and 43.3 percent screened positive for depression. In Canada, 10.5 percent of 3,969 nurses indicated suicidal ideation in the past year [245]. Younger nurses between 19 and 39 years old were more likely to report suicidal ideation than those over 40. Nurses in practice for over 10 years were less likely to report suicidal thoughts. In Europe, though samples sizes were smaller, a study of 385 female physicians in Sweden and 126 in Italy found 13.7 percent and 14.3 percent of physicians respectively reported suicidal thoughts in the past year [246]. 12 percent of male physicians, out of 456 from Sweden and 241 from Italy, indicated suicidal ideation [247]. European doctors and residents consistently show higher concerning rates of suicidal ideation than their North American counterparts [248]. Overall, suicidal ideation was encountered by 8.6 percent of 70,368 physicians per year. A survey in Australia indicated that 19 percent of medical students and 10 percent of physicians experienced suicidal thoughts within the past year. Four percent of medical students and 2 percent of doctors surveyed attempted suicide at any point in their lives [249]. Studying participants in real time, suicidal ideation increased, by the third month of internships by 4 times the frequency seen at the beginning of internship [250].

Get help

Depression

Physicians who died by suicide were less likely to have received any mental health treatment than suicides in the general population [251]. Therefore, it is not accurately known to what extent depression is prevalent among them. The prevalence of depression in nurses varies globally, but many studies have found the prevalence of depression among nurses to be higher than that of the general population [252].

In the US, in 2019, the prevalence of depression in adults over age 18, was found to be 7.8 percent [253]. Globally, the prevalence in adults over the age of 20 was found to be approximately 5 percent, or 280 million people [254]. Comparing physician rates of depression with those of the general population is difficult because of the greater stigma placed on physicians reporting depression. One study of general practice physicians in the UK found that male doctors suffered a higher prevalence of depression than the general UK population; women physicians were found to have a similar level of depression when compared to the sample population norms [255].

Levels of depression are higher in medical students and residents compared to the age matched general population [256]. One meta-analysis study of 129,123 medical students from 47 different countries found that overall, 27.2 percent of students had a prevalence of depression or depressive symptoms, but only 15.7 percent of those sought treatment [257]. A similar study of resident physicians found an overall prevalence of 28.8 percent of depression or depressive symptoms, percentages that increased from 20.9 percent to 43.2 percent with each year of training [258]. Similar findings were seen in doctor of pharmacy students; although research has been minimal, one study saw a 22 percent prevalence of depressive symptoms among students [259]. In nursing, a meta-analysis of 8,918 students found an overall depression of 34 percent, with higher prevalence seen in younger students [260].

There should be a greater approach to train all healthcare professionals and the general public on recognizing signs of depression, and signs of burnout in both ourselves and others.

Barriers to Obtaining Help for Burnout or Depression

It's clear to me from these studies, that the challenges of burnout and depression start early in medical training; intervention and awareness must be started early in medical training as well, while also continuing through all levels of education. In Australia, 56 percent of medical students and 64 percent of physicians indicated that they sought treatment for depression. Those accessing treatment were more females than males [261].

In the US, 64 percent of physicians who experienced suicidal ideation in the past year said they would get help [262]. Far fewer US medical students in the US sought help than those from Australia. For students who screened positive for depression, only 22 percent of them sought help through mental health services, and for those with suicidal ideation only 42 percent had treatment [263].

The top 3 barriers that were mentioned for seeking help were a lack of time, poor confidentiality, and stigma.

High stress among healthcare workers is normalized. Certain aspects of the career, such as long hours resulting in sleep deprivation, are seen as honorable indications of commitment. This stoicism produces competition among our peers instead of support and concern. It is quite common for physicians, who are so well apt at recognizing distress in patients, to fail at recognizing the same mental health concerns in themselves or in their peers.

Students beginning medical school have similar levels of depression, burnout, and quality of life (sometimes better) than those of other college graduates; but soon their levels of burnout and suicidality exceeded others [264].

Interestingly, research has not seen a significant difference in the depression of nursing students and that of non-nursing students [265]. There is an inherent risk within the organizational structure of medical training which has demonstrated to be cohesive for burnout and depression, which can coexist. Burnout can likely contribute to developing depression in those who are at a high risk for depression [266].

Burnout is seen in many professions within healthcare: nursing staff, allied workers, and pharmacists to name a few. However, the culture of medicine lends itself to burnout. It is a discipline with a zero-tolerance for making mistakes. This standard is often emphasized for people going into medicine, who often themselves tend towards perfectionism.

STUDENTS BEGINNING MEDICAL SCHOOL HAVE SIMILAR LEVELS OF DEPRESSION, BURNOUT, AND QUALITY OF LIFE THAN THOSE OF OTHER COLLEGE GRADUATES; BUT SOON THEIR LEVELS OF BURNOUT AND SUICIDALITY EXCEEDED OTHERS.

Suicide Risks

In a meta-analysis, male physicians had a 26 percent higher suicide risk than the general population, and for female physicians the risk of suicide was more than twice that of the general population, 146 percent higher [267]. These higher rates have been confirmed throughout multiple studies [268]. Risk factors for suicide include mental illness, substance use disorders, hopelessness, lack of support, chronic medical disorders, and previous suicide attempts [269]. Female physicians also evidenced a greater rate of alcohol abuse than women in the general population, although alcohol abuse is not the only risk factor [270].

To summarize, rates of suicide and burnout are higher in physicians than the general working population [271]. Now, this is not to say that physicians and healthcare providers have the highest risk of any profession in the United States [272], but as you can see from the figures alone, the need for change is still a grave concern affecting the lives of many.

Suicide Risk and Medical Specialty

Physicians are less likely to die of common medical conditions and causes than the general population [273]. Compare suicide statistics, however, and the story changes! In the general US population, suicide was the tenth leading cause of death in 2018 statistics; among resident physicians, suicide is the second leading cause of death [274]. For practicing physicians, a study reviewing causes of death in 1990 found that white males and female physicians were more likely to die from suicide than the general population; it was third highest cause of death. For black physicians, suicide rates did not differ from the general population [275].

Are there certain specialty areas within medicine that have a higher risk for suicide than others? It seems the statistics are higher for those providing frontline care, family medicine, general internal medicine, emergency medicine, and neurology [276]. Psychiatry, anesthesiology, and general surgery were also found to be high risk in another study [277].

Some studies looked at possible reasons behind the increased levels of burnout in anesthesiologists in particular [278]. Anesthesiologists are fairly isolated, especially when in the operating room, from consulting, discussing, or collaborating with peers. Staffing in the operating room usually doesn't have a backup if a physician were to need to reflect due to a challenging or adverse situation during surgery. Anesthesiologists are also particularly vulnerable under duress because they have easier access to drugs of abuse, or which could be used in suicide.

In a Canadian survey of physicians, surgical specialists had 74 percent greater odds of reporting low emotional well-being [279].

Estimated Rates of Physician Death by Suicide

An estimated 300–400 physicians die in the United States each year of suicide, a number equal to the size of a small medical school each year [280]. That estimate hasn't been truly updated since 1977 and does not reflect today's figure, so it is likely that the rates have changed along with the increased suicide rate in the general population. Due to the stigma and sensitivity attached to physician suicide, it's questionable whether all suicides are documented or listed as a different cause of death. The stigma attached to mental health and depression issues is especially high for health professionals. As discussed in depth in Section 2, it's problematic for physicians to seek professional help when they will be required to disclose past mental health history to their licensing boards. A diagnosis of depression is interpreted as detrimental, and in some state regulations, becomes a per-

AN ESTIMATED 300–400 PHYSICIANS DIE IN THE UNITED STATES EACH YEAR OF SUICIDE, A NUMBER EQUAL TO THE SIZE OF A SMALL MEDICAL SCHOOL EACH YEAR. THAT ESTIMATE HASN'T BEEN TRULY UPDATED SINCE 1977 AND DOES NOT REFLECT TODAY'S FIGURE.

manent part of the physician's professional record. That, and the potential for misdiagnosis when experiencing burnout, are some of the reasons many don't seek help. The public focus needs to be on addressing burnout and shifted to improving how the healthcare organizational system can better promote overall wellbeing and provide an atmosphere where seeking help is promoted and caring interventions are established to prevent burnout.

Substance Use and Burnout

Interestingly, physicians in the specialties found to experience higher rates of burnout are also treated more frequently for addiction/substance use disorders, although a 2015 survey showed the prevalence of substance use disorders in physicians is close to that of the general American population (15.4 percent vs. 12.6 percent respectively) [281].

From the Canadian Society of Addiction Medicine, addiction is defined as a "chronic disease of brain reward, motivation, memory, and related circuitry. Dysfunction in these circuits leads to characteristic biological, psychological, social and spiritual manifestations" [282].

In a study of physicians being treated for addictions, otherwise known as substance-use disorders – at 16 state physician health programs in the United States, over 50 percent of physicians were in the specialties of family medicine (20%), internal medicine (13%), anesthesiology (11%), emergency medicine (7%), and psychiatry (7%). Alcohol was the most common substance being used (50%), followed by opiates (36%), intravenous drugs (14%), and then stimulants (8%) [283].

Anaesthesiologists, according to some studies, have over twice the rate of substance use disorders that physicians in other specialties have [284]. Alcohol was again found to be the most used substance.

Physicians seem to be more affected than the general public when it comes to alcohol use disorders, with female physicians showing a higher percentage (21.4%) than males (12.9%) [285]. The majority of alcohol use disorders in the general population (from 2018 data) occur in those aged 18 to 25 years old (10.1%); however, 5.1 percent of people over 26 years old abuse alcohol [286]. Substance use disorders must be managed by physicians in the same way they are in the general population. They need to be identified, diagnosed, and treated with on-going follow-up. Oftentimes, co-workers and colleagues are the first to be aware of and identify the issue, since physicians are often unlikely to seek out help on their own [287]).

Physician health programs (PHP's) are available to help doctors with these disorders [288]. These groups aim to protect patients and save the life and career of physicians with a substance use disorder. These PHP's can be very effective treatment programs with promising success rates. Instead of immediate disciplinary actions from regulatory bodies or employing organizations, compliance with the PHPs guidance for treatment and monitoring usually leads to successful outcomes for the physician who will submit to it. A physician who fails to comply with the program's direction would require referral of that physician to the regulatory body [289]. The Ontario Medical Association Physician Health Program reported that 85 percent of physicians successfully complete 5 years of monitoring for moderate to severe substance use disorder, and of those physicians, 71 percent never use again [290]. These results are great news and demonstrate much better success rates than the general population, which is 40-60 percent.

Burnout Risk and Practice Setting

For physicians, the risk of burnout can also vary between practice settings. In the US, those in private practice have shown to be at a higher risk than those in academic settings [291]. A 2017 survey in Canada revealed that physicians in a hospital setting as opposed to private office/clinic, academic setting, or an administrative corporate office, had greater odds of incurring low emotional, social, and psychological well-being at 48 percent, 30 percent, and 39 percent respectively [292].

Impact of Gender and Age on Burnout Risk

Gender and age can influence a significant difference in risk factors for burnout as well. Younger workers show a higher risk of burnout, as do females in comparison to both older professionals and their male counterparts [293]. It could be as some believe that the younger generation is somewhat less equipped to handle the imbalances of occupational pressure and stressors and their personal capabilities, leading to burnout. I want to point out, however, that they are experiencing pressures today that were unknown before as the professions of medicine have change, especially in the area of technology.

Each change in the industry may hold its own advantages and disadvantages. Today's healthcare workers have added time constraints and performance measures that did not exist in previous generations. Patients have greater input into their own care; in the past, patients considered a physician's recommendation as definitive expert advice, but now, patients can conduct their own online research prior to an appointment, bringing with them many more questions or discussion points for the physician. That, plus new government and insurance-related regulations, make it more difficult for physicians to manage the allotted time.

Patients have varied expectations on how male versus female physicians will interact during their visit. Female patients often associate being listened to as an indication of receiving empathetic care [294]. Female physicians tend to ask more psychosocial questions during appointments which increases their appointment durations 10 percent longer than male physicians [295]. In an experiment, female patients were likely to base their rating of satisfaction with a female physician on how caring the communication style was, yet style of communication did not impact their satisfaction rating for a male physician [296].

> **YOUNGER WORKERS SHOW A HIGHER RISK OF BURNOUT, AS DO FEMALES IN COMPARISON TO BOTH OLDER PROFESSIONALS AND THEIR MALE COUNTERPARTS.**

If a female physician expressed uncertainty to a male patient about their diagnosis, the problem origins, or its best treatment, they'd give the female physician a lower patient satisfaction rating; if a male physician expressed uncertainty, satisfaction ratings from male patients were unaffected [297].

These kind of gender expectations may offer some insight as to the gender differences that are also witnessed in cases of burnout, which affects female physicians at a higher rate. Female physicians feel less control when it comes to their work, their schedules, their volume of patients, or their medical opinion about length of hospital stays. Additionally, studies show that every increase in working hours by 5 hours over a 40 hour week, adds 12 to 15 percent to a female physician's risk of burnout [298].

Female physicians often must work harder to prove themselves in workplaces where biases are present, yet they are often paid less than their male counterparts [299]. One study looked at the salary of over 10,000 academic physicians in public United States medical schools and found that female physicians earned 8 percent less ($19,879 USD) than males, even after accounting for age, experience, faculty rank, research and other potential factors [300]. The Association of Medical Colleges had similar findings when they conducted their first report on salary equity in 2019 [301].

The report in 2021 includes analysis of compensation by race/ethnicity. Of the 154 participating medical schools in the US, gender and race or ethnicity was reported for 98,406 full-time faculty along with the other variables. Frequently, white men received higher compensation than women of any race/ethnicity and men of other races/ethnicities, and white women were sometimes compensated more than women of color. Pay inequities have not seen much change, and gender remains the main influence in pay inequity, even in departments where women were in the majority among faculty.

IF A FEMALE PHYSICIAN EXPRESSED UNCERTAINTY TO A MALE PATIENT ABOUT THEIR DIAGNOSIS, THE PROBLEM ORIGINS, OR ITS BEST TREATMENT, THEY'D GIVE THE FEMALE PHYSICIAN A LOWER PATIENT SATISFACTION RATING; IF A MALE PHYSICIAN EXPRESSED UNCERTAINTY, SATISFACTION RATINGS FROM MALE PATIENTS WERE UNAFFECTED.

My search for data on the impact of work and family conflicts on burnout risk for female physicians has been inconclusive. Risks for burnout don't seem to vary whether female physicians have no children versus multiple children; however, some studies show lower burnout occurs when there is support for work-life balance provided by organizations, colleagues, and/or a spouse or a significant other. That decrease in burnout was documented from a survey of women under 45 years old [302].

Change Is Needed to Prevent Burnout

Education regarding burnout needs to expand so that blame is no longer placed on individuals who fall victim to this common occupational hazard. Society can also be involved, by holding healthcare organizations accountable, and ultimately advocating for these improvements.

The contributing factors and consequences of burnout are clear, but the necessary action, which moves research to real-world application and improves the overall healthcare system, is not. Healthcare organizations should begin facing the factors that contribute to burnout and decide how they can and will address these factors to improve workplace conditions. Hospitals, clinics, training programs, and healthcare corporations need to be accountable for implementing changes that lift the burdens currently placed on healthcare professionals and improve the resources that are available to them. Strategies are discussed in section 8.

Occupational Hazard within Healthcare

Physicians often miss out on living the healthy life they aim to instill or empower in their patients, too often succumbing to the occupational hazards of burnout and its related ailments. These hazards are not common knowledge when considering a career in healthcare, and it's not that the information can't be found if you seek it out either. While medical schools, residency programs, and hospitals promote 'wellness programs' and various health strategies under the premise of self-care or mental wellbeing, this is often done without providing underlying information regarding the threat burnout will be to its professionals and the importance of not taking this threat lightly.

Self-care and wellness programs can be powerful tools for wellness, but there are factors that increase the risk of burnout which cannot be addressed simply through wellness, exercise, or mindfulness. Do companies assess changes in burnout or wellness before, during, and after these programs? You cannot truly know how effective programs are, or what components in combination are best to improve engagement, without some honest and thorough evaluation.

The statistics on burnout do not seem to be changing. That should get the attention of our healthcare leadership! Wellness programs must not be enough, and research has shown that more effective methods must be utilized to significantly cut overall burnout [303]. Widespread discussion needs to take place, not only among healthcare professionals, but within the organizations, because many factors causing burnout are organizational, job-related factors which are outside of an individual's control.

The Role of Healthcare Organizations

Healthcare organizations and the work environment they create or allow play a huge role in burnout, but the majority of publications discussing these issues don't often address them as potential agents of change. Articles on burnout in medical journals and medical association publications generally target and address the healthcare professionals on a personal level. The target for

AWARENESS THROUGHOUT SOCIETY IS NEEDED CONCERNING THE IMPACT BURNOUT IS HAVING ON THE ENTIRE HEALTHCARE SYSTEM; IN ONE FORM OR ANOTHER, WE HAVE ALL CONTRIBUTED TO THE BURNOUT, WHETHER ACTIVELY OR IN COMPLACENCY, AND SO WE MUST ALL BEGIN TO CONTRIBUTE TO THE WELL-BEING OF OUR HEALTHCARE WORKERS!

potential change is aimed at the level of the individual, rather than the organizations.

To combat the burnout epidemic, there needs to be widespread public concern that doesn't restrict the discussion to only healthcare personnel. It's not a new issue, but a societal one that involves multiple players within the work system, including the patient, the public consumer. Awareness throughout society is needed concerning the impact burnout is having on the entire healthcare system; in one form or another, we have all contributed to the burnout, whether actively or in complacency, and so we must all begin to contribute to the well-being of our healthcare workers!

The Time to Start Is Now

The recent, and likely to be recurrent, Coronavirus pandemic has only made it more imperative that we start now to tackle the issue of burnout. As the viral pandemic wanes, the pandemic of burnout is becoming highly evident. All the Pre-COVID-19 burdens will be added to by the COVID-era burdens of an entirely overwhelmed healthcare system, lack of resources, and personnel and facility shortages.

In Section 2, burnout was discussed in the context of Maslow's Hierarchy. The application of the pandemic to that discussion are immense. Shortages of staff and personal protective equipment (PPE) are causing personnel to be overworked and seriously and morally distressed.

Moral distress was rampant during the pandemic. Healthcare professionals voiced their concerns for the lack of PPE; they faced a moral dilemma as they worked to save the lives of their patients while at times sacrificing their own safety and the safety of their families due to the lack of adequate protection [304]. This study identified common areas of concern and sources of anxiety for healthcare workers in the pandemic [305]:

- Delayed access to testing for COVID-19 if symptoms develop.
- Access to childcare as work hours increased and schools were closed.
- Ability to provide support for needs such as food, housing, and transportation as their work demands increased.
- Worry about the lack of communication and accurate, current information on a pandemic in which knowledge was in infancy.
- Providing competent care if required to work in a new area they are not specialized in, for example the intensive care unit.

Eventually, when lifesaving clinical resources become sparse, clinicians are faced with another dilemma: to decide between patients that need these scarce resources; decisions like that could mean deciding between life or death for a patient.

These mentally anguishing scenarios are a recipe for burnout. If it continues, I anticipate many healthcare professionals will either be leaving their jobs or will be required to, due to illness. The healthcare system will see a personnel shortage and increased expenses. This is already happening and is only projected to worsen.

One Canadian study conducted a survey between August and October 2020 and found a prevalence of burnout in 68 percent of the physicians who responded [306]. Interestingly, high rates of burnout did not differ significantly between physicians that cared for patients with COVID-19, and those who did not provide direct care. That tells me that the pandemic's effects have been far reaching.

One study showed that if a physician knew someone diagnosed with COVID-19, or someone who died from a COVID-19 infection, then that physician was much more likely to screen positive for depression, stress, anxiety, and post-traumatic stress disorder [307].

Twenty-one percent of those surveyed, indicated that they either planned to quit a job position or had already quit a position [308]. Forty-one percent also indicated that they had a poor work-life balance, with less personal or family time outside of work. Considering that not all burned out health professionals will leave, those who stay may suffer in silence, reflecting the exhaustion, cynicism, and reduced personal accomplishment, that are hallmarks of burnout. Other possible consequences of burnout for those that stay include poor health, potential workplace injuries, and possibly suicidal ideation. Patient care will eventually suffer as this mountain of symptoms lands on burned out physicians and other healthcare workers.

Key Chapter Points

- There is an inherent risk within the organizational structure of medical training which has demonstrated to be conducive to burnout and depression.
- Rates of suicide and burnout are higher in physicians than many in the general working population.
- Female physicians have higher suicide rates than the general population and higher risk than their male counterparts.
- Estimated number of physicians dying in the United States is likely more than 300-400 physicians per year, or one per day which was estimated in 1977.

Get help

SECTION 5:

The Consequences of Burnout for the Patient

For patients on the receiving end of care from burned out health care personnel, they can become unfortunate cases linked to medical errors. If personnel are disengaged, the resulting poor communication can cause a bad experience for patients who are unwell and in need of care, and potentially grave consequences.

CHAPTER 15:
MEDICAL ERRORS AND DISENGAGED PERSONNEL

"I am reluctant to go in for care...I'm tired of being handled like an ugly bag of mostly water."

Goals: Understand the impact of burnout on medical errors and patient safety.

The World Health Organization (WHO) estimates that for every 1 out of 300 patients, there is a risk of death due to a medical accident [309]. The WHO stated that the healthcare industry has a poor safety record in comparison to other industries such as the aviation or nuclear industries. In aviation, for instance, the risk to travelers dying in an airplane is 1 in 3 million [310].

One such study believes that many errors are likely missed, especially those resulting in death, since there was no true coding method that might indicate a cause of death due to error [311]. The cause of death that is noted on a death certificate is designated by a code from the International Classification of Disease (ICD) which is created and maintained through the WHO. Under the now-superseded ICD Version 10, most forms of error be it human error or systemic at root, would not be registered.

According to the World Health Organization, at least 117 countries utilize the ICD codes as a method to record their mortality data [312]. Since regulations in 1967, all of the Member States of the WHO are expected to use the most current ICD as means of reporting and monitoring death and disease. This helps with the widespread collection and dissemination of data for evidence-based decision-making and analysis. However, it can be argued that the stigma needs to be removed from accurately reporting cases of error – as it would be easier to analyze all the data on medical errors as a cause of death and make necessary changes to avoid similar errors in the future [313].

It was suggested that another field on the death certificates be added to indicate whether the patient's death was attributed to a preventable complication during care [314]. The 11th edition of the International Classification for Disease recently added additional safety issues under the heading 'causes of healthcare related harm or injury', which were implemented in 2022 [315]. As countries gradually implement the ICD Version 11, these changes could aid future research, and with widespread use of the new coding infrastructure, data regarding medical errors can be captured.

A Global Phenomenon

Mandatory and voluntary event reporting usually takes place for healthcare adverse events. When considering the United States, the form of reporting differs between each state and usually between various healthcare organizations [316]. In 2009, the World Health Organization developed a framework to organize and define patient safety concepts in the Conceptual Framework for the International Classification for Patient Safety (ICPS) [317]. The framework would allow the study, analysis, and comparison of safety data worldwide and across multiple disciplines.

In 2000, a national report on medical errors in the US health care system estimated that medical errors were responsible for 44,000 to 98,000 deaths. The estimate of 44,000 was generated by using the data from a study completed on adverse medical events occurring in Colorado and Utah in 1992, and the higher estimate of 98,000 was extrapolated from the results of a study in New York conducted in 1984 [318]. In 2016, another group of researchers estimated that deaths due to medical error were closer to over 200,000 deaths per year, which they claimed would make it the third leading cause of death in the US [319]. While the methodology and validity of these estimates is questionable (especially since one study considered errors made near the time of death, errors which weren't necessarily the cause of death), the figures they estimated were staggering [320].

In Canada, excluding Quebec, a retrospective data review in 2014-2015, found that 5.6 percent of hospitalizations, amounting to 138,000 patients or 1 in 18, had at least one "harmful event" occur during care, defined as potentially preventable harm [321]. In those patients who had a harmful event occur, 12.5 percent died, or 1 in 8, although causation is unknown. Compared to the leading causes of death in Canada, 17,300 patient deaths would equate to the third leading cause of death after cancer and heart disease [322].

The UK's National Health Service (NHS) estimated that between 300,000 and 1.4 million negative or adverse medical events happened in the year 2000 alone, averaging approximately 850,000 a year: that's 10 percent of the 8.5 million patients admitted each year [323]. Of these 850,000 incidents, 65 percent were considered preventable or 'near misses,' with thankfully less than 1 percent involving serious harm, and less than 0.5 percent were associated with death [324]. The number of deaths, likely an underestimate, would be approximately 3,500 patients.

In Australia, a study of over 14,000 patient charts in 28 hospitals found that 16.6 percent likely had an adverse event occur, half of which may

have been preventable [325]. Almost 14 percent of those adverse events resulted in patients suffering permanent disability and 4.9 percent died,
although the deaths may not have been caused by the adverse event itself
[326].

Global estimates predict that medical error contributes to patient harm,
overall patient harm ranks 14th as a cause of illness or death worldwide
[327].

Studies of hospital-acquired conditions also have accuracy-related limitations; patients may not die because of the adverse event or acquired
condition, but rather they may die with it [328]. For example, a patient may
contract a bacterial infection during a hospital stay due to failure in clinical management; it may be difficult to determine however, when this
hospital-acquired bacterial infection in and of itself raised the risk of the
patient's death. Did they die due to the infection or from their underlying illness? Studies and reports also can't easily distinguish how such
infections were acquired by the patient; not all infections occurring in
hospitals are necessarily caused by healthcare personnel or poor clinical
management. So, with that said, it's difficult to draw very exact conclusions looking back at patient records. Instead, if a review of the error is
made at the time of death the details and factors involved in that specific
event can be better understood.

Defining Medical Errors

To adequately discuss burnout as it contributes to medial errors, I must
point out that even the term 'medical error' in itself is not consistently or
uniformly defined in medical research. Since the report on error by the
Institute of Medicine in 2000, definitions have not been uniform, and
the methods to record the death certificate itself has not changed. If the

issue of medical error reporting is to be accurately recorded for national and international comparison and research, then a more accurate way to capture this information should be adapted worldwide. Widespread recognition and use of the ICD Version 11 and its updated codes would assist our profession greatly in uniformly tracking errors worldwide.

Patient Safety

The WHO started a global patient safety program in 2004. They developed a list of terms in 2009 to create uniformity in the international discussion of adverse medical events called the International Classification for Patient Safety [329]. It may not have widespread use yet, as there is much variation in definitions within research on patient safety and adverse events, but they published in 2016 a basic outline of the information needed for incident reporting, called the Minimal Information Model for Patient Safety Incident Reporting and Learning Systems. When reporting is uniform and done so on a large scale, it will be easier to identify possible trends and strategize improvements to reduce both the incidence of errors and adverse events.

Key Chapter Points

- For every 1 out of 300 patients there is a risk of death due to a medical accident.
- If the issue of medical error reporting is to be accurately recorded for national and international comparison including research, then an accurate way to capture this information should be adapted worldwide.

- It is estimated that globally medical error would equate to the 14th leading cause of illness or death. In some countries, this calculation is higher.
- When reporting is uniform and done on a large scale it will be easier to identify possible trends and structure improvements.

SECTION 6:

Consequences of Burnout for the Healthcare Organization

For healthcare organizations, loss of personnel can cost up to billions of dollars in high rates of staff turnover and training costs. Unhappy staff and patients, increased risk of malpractice suits, and decreased referrals can all stem from burnout.

CHAPTER 16:
UNDERSTANDING THE
COSTS OF BURNOUT

*"The immense burden of burnout demands a new
level of transparency by organizations to rectify it."*

Goals: Prioritize burnout prevention within the company framework.

Why is burnout a societal issue and not just a personal one? Burnout leads to compromises in professionalism and thus healthcare, errors become more prevalent, and the lines of communication fray, reducing patient satisfaction and undermining the integrity of the healthcare system [330]. A survey of thousands of patients and nurses in hospitals across 12 European countries and the US, found that patients felt unsatisfied with hospitals that also had a high percentage of nurses who said they were burned out [331]. Physicians' levels of burnout are also connected to lower patient satisfaction [332].

As the healthcare system suffers, ultimately the patients suffer, and vice versa. Burnout is a primary reason that 2,400 physicians in the US leave medicine each year [333]. That turnover alone costs us $4.6 billion USD per year [334]. In Canada, the cost of burnout-related turnover was estimated at $213.1 million CAD in lost services [335], combining the cost of both early retirement and reduced clinic hours. These high economic costs don't even consider the added litigation risk, reduced quality of care, lower patient satisfaction which can lead to decreased referrals and the poor reputation of healthcare professionals in the community. The cost for nurse turnover has been estimated at $82, 000 - $88, 000 per nurse [336].

Burnout Classification Internationally

Burnout in and of itself, is another issue that is not classified consistently around the globe.

In North America, within the former International Classification of Diseases, Tenth Revision (ICD-10), burnout was classified under the category of 'problems related to life-management difficulty' and it's listed as a "state of vital exhaustion" [337]. In the ICD eleventh revision (ICD-11) released in 2018 and which took effect in 2022, the WHO defines burnout as an occupational syndrome and says that it "should not be applied to describe experiences in other areas of life"[338].

Burnout is listed as different than adjustment disorder, anxiety disorders, mood disorders such as depression, or disorders associated with stress [339]. Notably, burnout is not mentioned in the classification of mental disorders published by the American Psychiatric Association (APA), called the Diagnostic and Statistical Manual of Mental Disorders. So, should burnout be considered a medical diagnosis?

In Europe, the definition of burnout varies from nation to nation. In some European countries, burnout is considered a medical diagnosis as indicated in the ICD-10 [340]. However, calling burnout a form of *vital exhaustion* as the ICD-10 does, limits the diagnosis and subsequent treatment to only one branch of the syndrome. This ignores issues of cynicism, a reduced perception of work value, and personal accomplishment, which are distinct issues and difficulties people experience when dealing with others while burning out, and that also lead to undesirable outcomes. These common burnout dynamics go far beyond exhaustion [341]. In fact, cynicism alone might be very closely tied with the work environment, and a core part of burnout [342]. Along the same line, calling burnout "a state of vital exhaustion" lends itself to misdiagnosis again if you use only that symptom of exhaustion. In the Netherlands, the Royal Dutch Medical Association defines burnout as a subtype of adjustment disorder [343]. With that diagnosis available in Europe, people are able to access compensation and treatment. However, the United Kingdom and 13 other European countries do not currently recognize burnout as a diagnosis [344].

Perhaps North American leaders in the industry fear that if burnout was recognized as a diagnosis, there would be a surge of requests for disability coverage [345].

The failure to fully understand or recognize burnout limits the access our professionals have to treatment and leads to greater stigma and possible misdiagnoses of the condition as chronic fatigue or depression [346].

Suggested Recognition as an Occupational Syndrome

The current lack of support and stigma attached to physicians who might otherwise seek help with their struggles has led to a culture that is largely indifferent and silent on the issue. Society is not openly discussing healthcare professionals burning out, so few people are able to connect-the-dots and shift our focus to prevention. Professionalism and patient satisfaction will likely continue to plummet. It's often the individual employee's end result that is focused on, instead of our culture adopting a wider lens to understand how the person reached that point.

To address burnout, will require an understanding that this is a genuine workplace syndrome as indicated in the current ICD-11, a hazard of the medical practice. It's not a mental health diagnosis, and therefore should not be described as such nor should an individual be labeled. Recognizing burnout as an occupational syndrome would allow personnel to receive compensation and treatment, and more importantly, organizations would be much more motivated to assess and strive to reduce the levels of burnout in the workplace.

Suggested Monitoring within Healthcare Organizations

I believe that anonymous burnout questionnaires should be provided in and to a database that would be accessible for healthcare organizations to conduct further research and improve upon their current work systems. Providing transparent public access to the results will hold our healthcare organizations accountable. Organizations themselves should also assess the data and levels of burnout in their organizations. Indeed, mandating organizations to track this information would help them address and hold to an expected standard. Public access will allow researchers and society to see how interventions and improvement measures are working. Health professionals considering employment with an organization, and health consumers attending a facility, would also then have a tangible way to make an informed decision.

> **ANONYMOUS BURNOUT QUESTIONNAIRES SHOULD BE PROVIDED IN AND TO A DATABASE THAT WOULD BE ACCESSIBLE FOR HEALTHCARE ORGANIZATIONS TO CONDUCT FURTHER RESEARCH AND IMPROVE UPON THEIR CURRENT WORK SYSTEMS.**

Interventions to Reduce Burnout and Improve Organizational Flow

A 2018 study looked at how a workload intervention might work within primary care practices [347]. The organizations switched from a dyad practice system to a team-based system and then were compared to the control group clinics that did not change their workload system. The dyad system consisted of a clinician and certified medical assistant. The team-based system consisted of two clinicians and three clinical assistants that would take care of a panel of patients. The study assessed 112 physicians on their levels of burnout and compared them to the control group clinics who didn't change.

Three months after the changes were made, all dimensions of burnout improved; physicians found that their workload improved, they experienced less emotional exhaustion and felt more engaged and less impersonal. Six months into the team-based system, all physicians still maintained the feeling of improvement in the areas of emotional exhaustion and depersonalization. Unfortunately, their workload felt overwhelming again; the authors of the study found that there was an underlying trend in the organization to allow the workload to revert.

Another workload intervention was observed over a 5-year timeframe, which found similar improvements in burnout measures and increased organizational well-being [348]. They studied multiple sites within a primary care group of 32 internal medicine and family medicine physicians. The group met every quarter to seek input from physicians on what influenced their well-being; the study also measured well-being via validated instruments. One critical area they focused on was the physician's control over their work environments (including their schedule and balancing various interests such as teaching, research, or inpatient or outpatient care). The organizations also got feedback about the order and efficiency of the clinic, issues like adequate staffing, changes to the patient template to improve the length and mix of cases, and improvements to decrease turnover of support staff. The third focus of the intervention was to improve the satisfaction with clinical care, emphasizing discussion of clinical improvements over discussion of administrative issues, a priority made to reflect the deeper meaning in their work. The intervention added case presentations at staff meetings to focus on clinical improvements, and respected clinician time when it came to bereavement over patients. Overall, these interventions produced a marked decrease in emotional exhaustion and improved emotional connection and empathy in the workplace [349].

Example Intervention to Reduce Burnout, Organizational Cost, and Improve Healthcare Quality

Reid and colleagues reviewed the patient-centered medical home model as an intervention. It reduced clinician burnout and improved the health care quality and costs within primary care [350]. The medical home model had primary care physicians working in multidisciplinary teams with specialist support along with other health care personnel. They paid each physician on a salary basis instead of volume-based fee-for-service payments. The goal was to improve the relationships with patients, provide a comprehensive approach to address patient needs, and allow more time for coordinating the care. The health group hired more staff to decrease the patient load per physician from 2,300 to 1,800. On staff were medical assistants, licensed practical nurses (LPN), physician assistants or nurse practitioners, registered nurses, and clinical pharmacists. Standard visit times were adjusted 20 minutes per patient, to 30-minute visits. A team approach was adopted, tasks were distributed, and daily meetings were held with visuals to communicate issues and track performance for team planning. Not only did patients report better satisfaction with care, but staff also showed significant improvement in burnout measures. After two years of these interventions being taken, the average emotional exhaustion scores decreased by more than half – a profound difference! The negativity of depersonalization also decreased markedly. As a result of these intervention measures, patients in the new clinic model had 6 percent fewer clinic visits; however, they used messaging methods 80 percent more and telephone encounters 5 percent more. These forms of contact were promoted in the new model. Patients had 29 percent fewer visits to the emergency department or urgent care after twenty-one months of the new clinic model. Patient admissions to the hospital were also 6 percent less than patients in the control clinics after twenty-one months. There were costs to implement the changes made to the clinic infrastructure; the estimates of the return on the investments were $1.50 for every $1 spent on recruiting and hiring additional staff. Cost analysis also showed that there was a savings of $10.30 per patient, although the finding did not reach statistical significance [351].

These are but a few examples of how interventions have shown to be to be beneficial in the healthcare industry – not only to decrease burnout, but to address many areas that could be measured, such as patient satisfaction, decreased hospitalizations, and lower costs. The premise that hiring additional staff will increase expenses does not have to be the case, as overall the benefits will outweigh expenses. Organizations must also consider the prevention of losses from staff burnout, the cost of staff taking more time off to recover, the improved team communication and performance, and for those we serve, greater patient satisfaction.

Key Chapter Points

- Burnout has been described as a main reason leading to 2,400 physicians in the US leaving medicine each year. This reflects as an estimated cost of $4.6 billion USD per year due to turnover and decreased hours.
- The cost for nurse turnover has been estimated to be $82,000–$88,000 per nurse.
- Recognize burnout as an occupational syndrome and integrate assessments and interventions into the healthcare organization infrastructure.
- Interventions for burnout have shown to be to be beneficial. Not only do they decrease burnout, but additionally they improve patient satisfaction, decrease hospitalizations and overall costs.

CHAPTER 17:
THE COST OF ADVERSE EVENTS

"Deficiencies in safety damage trust in healthcare systems, institutions, and governing bodies."

Goals: Reduce adverse events and allocate funding towards preventative measures.

The cost of adverse events can vary depending on the event and the outcomes. In Canada, one analysis estimated the average cost of adverse events as $6,800 per patient [352]. In 2014-2015, the estimate of hospital costs from adverse events was 1 percent of the total hospital spending, equating to $685 million excluding any physician fees [353]. It is worth noting that $281 million of that was specifically from infections acquired while in hospital. These numbers don't take into consideration outpatient costs from follow up or re-admissions.

Another analysis estimated a cost of $2.75 billion Canadian (CAD) each year, which includes adverse events occurring in the hospital/acute care ($1.3 billion CAD) and home care ($1.45 billion CAD) settings. In a typical developed country, such as the 35 countries who are part of the Organization for Economic Co-operation and Development (OECD), the estimated cost of adverse events is approximately 15 percent of the hospital acute care costs, which is thought to be an underestimate [354]. In 2008, the US estimated total cost was near one trillion dollars US [355].

Adverse events can lead to increased hospital stays, which a British study found to amount to nearly 500,000 days per year across England [356]. This number was similar to the finding in Canada from 2014-2015 where patients who experienced an adverse event were estimated to spend more than 500,000 additional days in hospital. This equates to more than 1,600 beds each day [357]. The adverse events that have the greatest impact leading to longer hospital stays are pressure ulcers*, and venous thromboembolisms (VTE)** [358]. The increased number of days would equate to $21.3 million GBP [359].

These costs indicate that preventative measures would be much less expensive than the costs attributed to adverse events, whether considering preventative measures for pressure ulcers, VTE or others [360].

For example, between 59 percent and 75 percent of VTEs are developed in a healthcare facility [361]. Approximately 67 percent of the deaths that occur due to VTE occur in hospitals [362]. In 2010 in the US, the cost ranged between $5 - $26.5 billion USD that would amount to 4-6 percent of a public hospital's expenditure [363]. The estimated cost of evidence-based preventative measures against VTE was under $600 million USD per year.

Key Chapter Points

- The cost of adverse events can vary depending on the event and the outcomes. Some estimates place it at up to 1 trillion US dollars.
- Adverse events can lead to increased hospital stays.

---

* Pressure ulcer: an injury to the skin caused by prolonged pressure.

** VTE: venous thromboembolism, when a blood clot forms in a vein.

- Costs attributed to adverse events have shown to far outweigh the costs required to implement preventative measures.

SECTION 7:
Addressing Burnout on an Organizational Level

We have covered a great number of factors that impact burnout. Many of these occur at an organizational level. Organizations and training centers can increase engagement among their workers and students by assessing their shortcomings and implementing necessary changes. There are always areas for improvement.

CHAPTER 18:
SIX STRATEGIES TO ADDRESS BURNOUT

"The wellness of each person in the healthcare field matters, no one wants to feel like they're disposable."

Goals: Address burnout at multiple levels, including training centers and healthcare organizations. Involve all key stakeholders, including the public, in mitigation efforts.

All around us, lives are being lost and we are never told about it, in the very healthcare profession that we value, and the family members whom we love. It is time to push policy makers and organizations into action. A good place to start for policy makers is the summary of recommendations and suggestions from the National Academy of Sciences committee to combat burnout. This summary of recommendations can be found in their report and summarized in a journal article from some of the committee members [364].

The summary provided below is adapted from this and adjusted to reflect the discussion points that were made within this book.

Six Strategies to Address Burnout

1. Healthcare professionals

    a. Develop a positive work environment for healthcare personnel, a supportive and fair environment where concerns are respected and listened to and responded to in a timely manner.

    b. Clinician's autonomy and feedback should be respected.

c. Each person should be treated fairly in all respects including their right to equal pay without discrimination.

d. Support interdisciplinary teamwork and team building initiatives with enhanced communication.

e. Make sure each of the human needs are met, ensuring adequate time off between shifts, rest, nutrition, and relief breaks, to name a few. Provide staff education in these domains including the impact these have on performance.

f. Regularly survey the organization's level of burnout and job satisfaction using measures that anonymously assess the progress of interventions and maintenance of the appropriate environment.

g. Incorporate individual interventions promoting wellness, such as open discussion groups and wellness activities. Include measures to follow up on how effective these interventions are in achieving the desired goals for personnel well-being, analyze the results, and make adjustments as necessary.

h. Implement a reward system to support workers and recognize work efforts.

2. Trainees

a. Develop positive learning environments for trainees: a supportive and fair environment where concerns are respected and listened to and responded to in a timely manner.

b. Create an environment of wellness and remove the barriers for trainees to obtain help when needed. To do so, normalize meetings with health and wellness staff; assign mentors to support and meet with trainees on a regularly scheduled basis.

c. Trainee autonomy and feedback should be respected and developed.

d. Each person should be treated fairly in all respects including their right to equal pay without discrimination.

e. Create an opportunity for increased training positions and prioritize integrating unmatched medical graduates into the healthcare workforce. For those meeting credentialing requirements, eliminate barriers for physician trainees in terms of visa restrictions.

f. Develop and support interdisciplinary teamwork and team building initiatives with enhanced communication.

g. Make sure each of the human needs are met, ensuring adequate time off between shifts, rest, nutrition and relief breaks, to name a few. Provide trainees education in these domains including the impact these have on performance.

h. Provide instruction on burnout, fatigue, substance use, and how to recognize signs of mental health issues and substance use disorders in oneself or others.

i. Regularly survey trainees on burnout, using measures that anonymously assess progress of interventions and maintenance of the appropriate environment.

j. Incorporate individual interventions promoting wellness, such as open discussion groups, team building, and wellness activities. Include measures to follow up on how effective these interventions are in achieving the desired goals for personnel's well-being, analyze the results, and make adjustments as necessary.

3. Resources

a. Ensure sufficient resources and full staffing. Develop a relief roster for each discipline in case of extenuating circumstances or emergencies during a shift.

b. Reassess expenditures and ensure money is utilized where it is needed; adequate staffing should be high priority.

c. Decrease the administrative burden on physicians by reviewing policies or standardized procedures that need not be mandatory.

d. Review unnecessary accreditation laws and requirements that increase administrative burdens on healthcare personnel and reduce time for patient care.

e. Ensure that financial clinic goals are feasible or reasonable for the number of staff and patients present.

4. Technology

a. Improve integrated technology. Ensure that the electronic health record is not hindering patient care. Minimize pop-ups or alerts during clinic hours to reduce unnecessary interruptions.

b. Survey clinician technology users in order to improve workflow usability.

c. Integrate technology to improve patient outcomes and reduce administrative burdens; ensure review and trial of technology by clinicians for appropriate feedback.

5. Prioritize Research

a. Prioritize ongoing research into burnout and monitor the progress of changes made within the healthcare organizational systems.

b. Government and research institutions should provide adequate research funding.

c. Research those factors often seen with burnout, such as substance use disorders, adverse events, and suicide.

d. Conduct research using standardized recording approaches wherever possible, to allow comparisons globally.

6. Involve All Stakeholders

It is not only policy makers, clinicians, and healthcare workers who should be involved in the decision making for system interventions, but also the public needs to have input.

Though each country's healthcare system and structures are different, the issue of burnout in the industry is universal. Why not form a global taskforce to help make the widespread adjustments needed to address the issues present and communicated in this book? There is no system or country that is immune to the pandemic of burnout, as seen in the global research examples cited herein, of which there are many more.

CONCLUSION

"Burnout didn't develop overnight, so we can't expect this issue to be resolved overnight. Even more reason why we must start the motions of change now."

The main aim of this book is not to solve the inherent issues within healthcare all at once; indeed, these are widespread, multilayered systemic issues and the issue of burnout, is in particular, one that will take time and a conscious, concerted effort. The goal, instead, is to shed light on the critical pandemic that is taking over our healthcare system with very little public awareness. Much like the Coronavirus pandemic, this burnout pandemic within the health care system affects every person – from healthcare worker, to patient, to the people intricately involved in the lives of each. We cannot take our individual or collective health for granted.

In the midst of the viral pandemic, the world at large came to appreciate the value of health in a new light. During the COVID-19 pandemic, we often saw a commendable global public display of support for healthcare workers fighting to combat the disease and to treat the ill, all at a high risk to themselves. It's important that the public continue their rally of support in tangible ways. The information within this book can help the public, healthcare workers, students, and administrators gain a more comprehensive and insightful understanding of what is draining the healthcare system and dangerously tipping the balance of wellness and engagement to burnout.

With such a broad repository of knowledge, we have a foundation upon which to build meaningful change. Those pursuing a career in healthcare should use this book to understand the factors related to burnout that will affect them. Whether one is a healthcare professional, patient, administrator, or organization executive, we can each affect the healthcare system positively in the current roles we each play. Let's act as ambassadors for change, speaking out against excessive demands, lack of resources, and mistreatment or abuse. It is only when we all rally behind the same cause, that we can change the system day by day.

The COVID-19 pandemic has shown the world what the truly essential services are. When all our entertainment and distractions are stripped away, we are left with our loved ones and our health, or lack thereof. Now is the time for everyone to demonstrate that we truly value healthcare and the personnel who are working to provide it. Changes should reflect the right priorities, which are the health and safety of patients and optimized care. This priority is completely intertwined and dependent on the wellness of our personnel: physicians, nurses, pharmacists, and many allied staff members. It is this critical infrastructure, consisting of a healthy working team of dedicated people that is the most important thing, and needs to be nurtured. The time for change is now or never; there is no time to wait!

The suggestions provided in section 7 can also be extrapolated to multiple career disciplines to improve the standard for workers' well-being.

We each play a pivotal part and together we can effect change. Those working within the healthcare system and experiencing burnout or mental illness should anticipate that change is coming. With the increasing awareness, support for those who are struggling will also increase, and the public can grow in understanding the complex impact burnout has on worker well-being. To those who are feeling burnt out, I want to say that as a society, we are here for you to listen and to do what we can to help one another and in so doing, improve the entire healthcare system.

If you are overwhelmed and struggling, know that there is hope! Please continue to the resource pages online to explore supportive tools and find resources in your area.

Now that Reality has been truly Checked, and you have completed the book, know that this is just the beginning. If you are inspired to take further steps to create positive change, please connect with our growing network of online support. We offer resources like the *Reality Check Wellness Workbook* and the *Mindful Coloring Companion*, as well as speaking and consulting services to help individuals and organizations address burnout effectively.

We are also actively developing courses to help you become a certified Burnout Champion and gain additional tools for meaningful change. If you found this Reality Check to be helpful, become a part of the movement. Together we can make a difference in relieving workplace stress.

Become a champion against burnout!

APPENDIX I:

Theoretical Frameworks to Increase Psychological Fortitude and Resilience

Use this appendix as a quick reference to access the frameworks discussed in this book. Refer to it often to refresh your skills and remain resilient in times of conflict and when errors are made.

REMAIN RESILIENT IN CONFLICTING SCENARIOS

Goals: Utilize the framework in difficult scenarios requiring resilience.

The framework I described in this book provides tools in the form of questions, to ask ourselves in any scenario, to clarify our thought process and the best response. The three questions to ask when assessing how to respond in a situation are:

1. Is this an opinion or fact?
2. Does what they think change the reality of how I see myself?
3. Do I have anything to prove?

REMAIN RESILIENT IN THE PRESENCE OF ERRORS

Goals: Utilize the framework in difficult scenarios that result in errors or perceived error.

In the strategy framework I presented earlier in the book, you can ask a set of questions to yourself to help respond to the demise-reflex or hindsight bias.

1. Was the error I made done so with a malicious intent?
2. Have I changed a key approach or habit that used to produce positive outcomes?
3. What can I learn from this error or situation?

NOTES

Introduction

1 National Library of Medicine, "Greek Medicine," https://www.nlm.nih.gov/ hmd/greek/greek_oath.html.

Chapter 1. Relationship Strains

2 Engineering National Academies of Sciences, and Medicine; National Academy of Medicine; Committee on Systems Approaches to Improve Patient Care by Supporting Clinician Well-Being, "Taking Action against Clinician Burnout: A Systems Approach to Professional Well-Being," in Taking Action against Clinician Burnout: A Systems Approach to Professional Well-Being (Washington (DC): National Academies Press, 2019).

3 Ibid.

4 L. C. Garcia et al., "Burnout, Depression, Career Satisfaction, and Work-Life Integration by Physician Race/Ethnicity," JAMA Netw Open 3, no. 8 (2020).

5 Ibid.

6 C. P. West, T. D. Shanafelt, and J. C. Kolars, "Quality of Life, Burnout, Educational Debt, and Medical Knowledge among Internal Medicine Residents," JAMA 306, no. 9 (2011).

7 Canadian Medical Association, "Cma National Physician Health Survey," Canadian Medical Association, https://www.cma.ca/sites/default/ files/2018-11/nph-survey-e.pdf.

8 Ibid.

9 Ibid.

10 Ibid.

11 Pascale Carayon, "The Balance Theory and the Work System Model ... Twenty Years Later," International Journal of Human-Computer Interaction 25, no. 5 (2009).

12 S. Martins Pereira et al., "Compared to Palliative Care, Working in Intensive Care More Than Doubles the Chances of Burnout: Results from a Nationwide Comparative Study," PLoS One 11, no. 9 (2016); G. M. Jones et al., "Factors Associated with Burnout among Us Hospital Clinical Pharmacy Practitioners: Results of a Nationwide Pilot Survey," Hosp Pharm 52, no. 11 (2017); E. Read and H. K. Laschinger, "Correlates of New Graduate Nurses' Experiences of Workplace Mistreatment," J Nurs Adm 43, no. 4 (2013).

13 B. Li et al., "Group-Level Impact of Work Environment Dimensions on Burnout Experiences among Nurses: A Multivariate Multilevel Probit Model," Int J Nurs Stud 50, no. 2 (2013).

14 D. S. Havens, J. H. Gittell, and J. Vasey, "Impact of Relational Coordination on Nurse Job Satisfaction, Work Engagement and Burnout: Achieving the Quadruple Aim," J Nurs Adm 48, no. 3 (2018).

15 J.K. Burgoon, L.K. Guerrero, and V. Manusov, Nonverbal Communication (Routledge, 2016).

16 Merriam-Webster, "Resilience," Merriam-Webster.com Dictionary, https://www.merriam-webster.com/dictionary/resilience.

17 Laura Petitta, Lixin Jiang, and Charmine E.J. Härtel, "Emotional Contagion and Burnout among Nurses and Doctors: Do Joy and Anger from Different Sources of Stakeholders Matter?," Stress and Health 33, no. 4 (2017).

18 Havens, Gittell, and Vasey.

19 J. H. Gittell, M. Godfrey, and J. Thistlethwaite, "Interprofessional Collaborative Practice and Relational Coordination: Improving Healthcare through Relationships," J Interprof Care 27, no. 3 (2013).

Chapter 2. Work–Life Imbalance

20 B. G. Arndt et al., "Tethered to the Ehr: Primary Care Physician Workload Assessment Using Ehr Event Log Data and Time-Motion Observations," Ann Fam Med 15, no. 5 (2017).

21 D. M. Zulman, N. H. Shah, and A. Verghese, "Evolutionary Pressures on the Electronic Health Record: Caring for Complexity," JAMA 316, no. 9 (2016).

22 Ibid.

23 Ibid.

24 C. M. Kuhn and E. M. Flanagan, "Self-Care as a Professional Imperative: Physician Burnout, Depression, and Suicide," Can J Anaesth 64, no. 2 (2017).

25 T. D. Shanafelt et al., "Relationship between Clerical Burden and Characteristics of the Electronic Environment with Physician Burnout and Professional Satisfaction," Mayo Clin Proc 91, no. 7 (2016); E. R. Melnick et al., "The Association between Perceived Electronic Health Record Usability and Professional Burnout among Us Physicians," ibid.95, no. 3 (2020).

26 National Academies of Sciences.

27 I. Philibert et al., "New Requirements for Resident Duty Hours," JAMA 288, no. 9 (2002).no. 9 (2002

28 L. Goitein et al., "The Effects of Work-Hour Limitations on Resident Well-Being, Patient Care, and Education in an Internal Medicine Residency Program," Arch Intern Med 165, no. 22 (2005).

29 Ibid.

30 Kuhn and Flanagan.

31 L. Block et al., "In the Wake of the 2003 and 2011 Duty Hours Regulations, How Do Internal Medicine Interns Spend Their Time?," J Gen Intern Med 28, no. 8 (2013).

32 Ibid.

33 Merriam-Webster, "Empathy," Merriam-Webster.com Dictionary, https://www.merriam-webster.com/dictionary/empathy.

34 J.; Lamm Decety, C., "Empathy Versus Personal Distress: Recent Evidence from Social Neuroscience," in The Social Neuroscience of Empathy, ed. Jean; Ickes Decety, William (The MIT Press, 2009).

35 Merriam-Webster, "Compassion," Merriam-Webster.com Dictionary, https://www.merriam-webster.com/dictionary/compassion.

36 Sonja Lyubomirsky, Kennon M. Sheldon, and David Schkade, "Pursuing Happiness: The Architecture of Sustainable Change," Review of General Psychology 9, no. 2 (2005).

37 Christina Maslach, "The Client Role in Staff Burn-Out," Journal of Social Issues 34, no. 4 (1978).

38 Ibid.

39 E. Gleichgerrcht and J. Decety, "Empathy in Clinical Practice: How Individual Dispositions, Gender, and Experience Moderate Empathic Concern, Burnout, and Emotional Distress in Physicians," PLoS One 8, no. 4 (2013).

40 Maslach.

41 J. L. Halpern, "Beyond "Detached Concern": The Cognitive and Ethical Function of Emotions in Medical Practice" (Yale University, 1993).

42 Bettina Lampert and Jürgen Glaser, "Detached Concern in Client Interaction and Burnout," International Journal of Stress Management 25, no. 2 (2018); James J. Gross, "The Emerging Field of Emotion Regulation: An Integrative Review," Review of General Psychology 2, no. 3 (1998).

43 J. Halpern, From Detached Concern to Empathy: Humanizing Medical Practice (Oxford University Press, USA, 2001).

44 Lampert and Glaser.

45 Ibid.

46 Gleichgerrcht and Decety.

47 H. Wilkinson et al., "Examining the Relationship between Burnout and Empathy in Healthcare Professionals: A Systematic Review," Burn Res 6 (2017); H. von Harscher et al., "The Impact of Empathy on Burnout in Medical Students: New Findings," Psychol Health Med 23, no. 3 (2018); P. T. Lee et al., "Empathy and Burnout: A Study on Residents from a Singapore Institution," Singapore Med J 59, no. 1 (2018).

48 B.Y. Lee, "Time to Stop Labeling Physicians as Providers," Forbes, https://www.forbes.com/sites/brucelee/2019/05/05/time-to-stop-labeling-physicians-as-providers/.

49   Health Education England, "Advanced Practice," https://www.hee.nhs.uk/our-work/advanced-clinical-practice.

Chapter 3. The Search for Meaning

50   H. J. Tak, F. A. Curlin, and J. D. Yoon, "Association of Intrinsic Motivating Factors and Markers of Physician Well-Being: A National Physician Survey," J Gen Intern Med 32, no. 7 (2017); A. Ziedelis, "Perceived Calling and Work Engagement among Nurses," West J Nurs Res 41, no. 6 (2019).

51   C. H. Rushton et al., "Burnout and Resilience among Nurses Practicing in High-Intensity Settings," Am J Crit Care 24, no. 5 (2015); V. Rasmussen et al., "Burnout among Psychosocial Oncologists: An Application and Extension of the Effort-Reward Imbalance Model," Psychooncology 25, no. 2 (2016); Jones et al.

52   Ziedelis.

53   T. D. Shanafelt et al., "Career Fit and Burnout among Academic Faculty," Arch Intern Med 169, no. 10 (2009).

54   Ibid.

55   NHS Employers, "What We Do," https://www.nhsemployers.org/about-us/what-we-do.

56   «National Engagement Service,» https://www.nhsemployers.org/engagement-and-networks/nhs-employers-engagement-service.

57   "The Relationship between Staff Engagement and Patient Experience," https://www.nhsemployers.org/-/media/Employers/Publications/Staff-engagement/IES-NE-case-studies/Common-themes.pdf.

58   Ibid.

59   National Academies of Sciences.

60   J. H. McAbee et al., "Factors Associated with Career Satisfaction and Burnout among Us Neurosurgeons: Results of a Nationwide Survey," J Neurosurg 123, no. 1 (2015); West, Shanafelt, and Kolars; Dinah Wisenberg Brin, "Taking the Sting out of Medical School Debt," Association of American

Medical Colleges, https://www.aamc.org/news-insights/taking-sting-out-medical-school-debt.

61 K. Keeton et al., "Predictors of Physician Career Satisfaction, Work-Life Balance, and Burnout," Obstet Gynecol 109, no. 4 (2007); M. D. McHugh and C. Ma, "Wage, Work Environment, and Staffing: Effects on Nurse Outcomes," Policy Polit Nurs Pract 15, no. 3-4 (2014).

62 T. D. Shanafelt et al., "Burnout and Career Satisfaction among American Surgeons," Ann Surg 250, no. 3 (2009); T. D. Shanafelt et al., "Burnout and Career Satisfaction among Us Oncologists," J Clin Oncol 32, no. 7 (2014).

63 M. Pratt, M. Kerr, and C. Wong, "The Impact of Eri, Burnout, and Caring for Sars Patients on Hospital Nurses' Self-Reported Compliance with Infection Control," Can J Infect Control 24, no. 3 (2009); Jones et al.

64 McHugh and Ma.

Chapter 4. Neglected Needs and Ignored Personal Priorities

65 Association.

66 L. Kane, "Medscape National Physician Burnout & Suicide Report 2020: The Generational Divide," Medscape, https://www.medscape.com/slideshow/2020-lifestyle-burnout-6012460.

67 T. Locke, "Medscape Uk Doctors' Burnout & Lifestyle Survey 2020," Medscape, https://www.medscape.com/slideshow/uk-doctors-burnout-2020-6013312.

68 A. H. Maslow, "A Theory of Human Motivation," Psychological Review 50, no. 4 (1943).

69 D. E. Shapiro et al., "Beyond Burnout: A Physician Wellness Hierarchy Designed to Prioritize Interventions at the Systems Level," Am J Med 132, no. 5 (2019).

70 C. Maslach and M. P. Leiter, "Understanding the Burnout Experience: Recent Research and Its Implications for Psychiatry," World Psychiatry 15, no. 2 (2016).

71 Ibid.; B. Bakker Arnold and Evangelia Demerouti, "The Job Demands-Resources Model: State of the Art," Journal of Managerial Psychology 22, no. 3 (2007).

72 W.B. Schaufeli, C. Maslach, and T. Marek, Professional Burnout: Recent Developments in Theory and Research (Taylor & Francis, 2017).

73 M. Panagioti et al., "Controlled Interventions to Reduce Burnout in Physicians: A Systematic Review and Meta-Analysis," JAMA Intern Med 177, no. 2 (2017).

74 A. W. Solomon et al., "Urine Output on an Intensive Care Unit: Case-Control Study," BMJ 341 (2010).

75 D. M. Berwick, T. W. Nolan, and J. Whittington, "The Triple Aim: Care, Health, and Cost," Health Aff (Millwood) 27, no. 3 (2008).

76 T. Bodenheimer and C. Sinsky, "From Triple to Quadruple Aim: Care of the Patient Requires Care of the Provider," Ann Fam Med 12, no. 6 (2014).

77 L. R. Thomas, J. A. Ripp, and C. P. West, "Charter on Physician Well-Being," JAMA 319, no. 15 (2018).

78 Survey Coordination Centre, "2019 Nhs Staff Survey," National Health Service England, https://www.nhsstaffsurveyresults.com/wp-content/uploads/2020/01/P3255_ST19_National-briefing_FINAL_V2.pdf.

79 C. Rees et al., "The Effects of Occupational Violence on the Well-Being and Resilience of Nurses," J Nurs Adm 48, no. 9 (2018); J. Shi et al., "The Frequency of Patient-Initiated Violence and Its Psychological Impact on Physicians in China: A Cross-Sectional Study," PLoS One 10, no. 6 (2015); Syed Harris Laeeque et al., "How Patient-Perpetrated Workplace Violence Leads to Turnover Intention among Nurses: The Mediating Mechanism of Occupational Stress and Burnout," Journal of Aggression, Maltreatment & Trauma 27, no. 1 (2018); H. Kim et al., "Mediating Effects of Workplace Violence on the Relationships between Emotional Labour and Burnout among Clinical Nurses," J Adv Nurs 74, no. 10 (2018).

80   J. Jakobsson, M. Axelsson, and K. Ormon, "The Face of Workplace Violence: Experiences of Healthcare Professionals in Surgical Hospital Wards," Nurs Res Pract 2020 (2020).

81   Shi et al.

82   Ibid.

83   Rees et al.

84   X. Duan et al., "The Impact of Workplace Violence on Job Satisfaction, Job Burnout, and Turnover Intention: The Mediating Role of Social Support," Health Qual Life Outcomes 17, no. 1 (2019).

85   National Institute for Occupational Safety and Health (NIOSH), "Occupational Health Safety Network (Ohsn)," Centers for Disease Control and Prevention, https://www.cdc.gov/niosh/topics/ohsn/.

86   M. R. Groenewold et al., "Workplace Violence Injury in 106 Us Hospitals Participating in the Occupational Health Safety Network (Ohsn), 2012-2015," Am J Ind Med 61, no. 2 (2018).

87   S. T. Noland et al., "Analysis of Career Stage, Gender, and Personality and Workplace Violence in a 20-Year Nationwide Cohort of Physicians in Norway," JAMA Netw Open 4, no. 6 (2021); J. P. Phillips, "Workplace Violence against Health Care Workers in the United States," N Engl J Med 374, no. 17 (2016).

88   Jakobsson, Axelsson, and Ormon.

89   K. L. Edward et al., "A Systematic Review and Meta-Analysis of Factors That Relate to Aggression Perpetrated against Nurses by Patients/Relatives or Staff," J Clin Nurs 25, no. 3-4 (2016).

90   D. Acquadro Maran et al., "Gender Differences in Reporting Workplace Violence: A Qualitative Analysis of Administrative Records of Violent Episodes Experienced by Healthcare Workers in a Large Public Italian Hospital," BMJ Open 9, no. 11 (2019); Y. Kobayashi et al., "Workplace Violence and Its Effects on Burnout and Secondary Traumatic Stress among Mental Healthcare Nurses in Japan," Int J Environ Res Public Health 17, no. 8 (2020).

91 M. Li et al., "The Relationship of Workplace Violence and Nurse Outcomes: Gender Difference Study on a Propensity Score Matched Sample," J Adv Nurs 76, no. 2 (2020); Noland et al.

92 Noland et al.

93 L. Shi et al., "Prevalence and Correlates of Symptoms of Post-Traumatic Stress Disorder among Chinese Healthcare Workers Exposed to Physical Violence: A Cross-Sectional Study," BMJ Open 7, no. 7 (2017).

94 F. Havaei, M. MacPhee, and S. E. Lee, "The Effect of Violence Prevention Strategies on Perceptions of Workplace Safety: A Study of Medical-Surgical and Mental Health Nurses," J Adv Nurs 75, no. 8 (2019).

95 WorkSafeBC, "Health Care and Social Services High Risk Strategy," https://www.worksafebc.com/en/about-us/what-we-do/high-risk-strategies/health-care.

96 National Institute for Occupational Safety and Health (NIOSH), "Occupational Violence Fast Facts," Centers for Disease Control and Prevention, https://www.cdc.gov/niosh/topics/violence/fastfacts.html.

97 Havaei, MacPhee, and Lee.

98 Ibid.

99 Duan et al; Paula Brough, "Workplace Violence Experienced by Paramedics: Relationships with Social Support, Job Satisfaction, and Psychological Strain," Australas. J. Disast. Trauma Stud. 2 (2005).

Chapter 5. Racial and Ethnic Bias

100 American Association of Medical Colleges, "Figure 18. Percentage of All Active Physicians by Race/Ethnicity, 2018," https://www.aamc.org/data-reports/workforce/interactive-data/figure-18-percentage-all-active-physicians-race/ethnicity-2018.

101 M. Walji, "Diversity in Medical Education: Data Drought and Socioeconomic Barriers," CMAJ 187, no. 1 (2015).

102 Merriam-Webster, "Stereotype," Merriam-Webster.com Dictionary, https://www.merriam-webster.com/dictionary/stereotype.

103 L. Quillian et al., "Do Some Countries Discriminate More Than Others? Evidence from 97 Field Experiments of Racial Discrimination in Hiring," Sociological Science 6, no. 18 (2019).

104 Project Implicit, "Project Implicit," https://implicit.harvard.edu/implicit/.

Chapter 6. Gender Bias

105 Merriam-Webster, "Overachiever," Merriam-Webster.com Dictionary, https://www.merriam-webster.com/dictionary/overachiever.

106 "Proof," Merriam-Webster.com Dictionary, https://www.merriam-webster.com/dictionary/proof.

107 Christina Maslach, "Finding Solutions to the Problem of Burnout," Consulting Psychology Journal: Practice and Research 69, no. 2 (2017).

Chapter 7. Unrealistic Expectations

108 L. M. Carpenter, A. J. Swerdlow, and N. T. Fear, "Mortality of Doctors in Different Specialties: Findings from a Cohort of 20000 Nhs Hospital Consultants," Occup Environ Med 54, no. 6 (1997); D. T. Ko et al., "Comparison of Cardiovascular Risk Factors and Outcomes among Practicing Physicians Vs the General Population in Ontario, Canada," JAMA Netw Open 2, no. 11 (2019).

109 N. A. Ali et al., "Continuity of Care in Intensive Care Units: A Cluster-Randomized Trial of Intensivist Staffing," Am J Respir Crit Care Med 184, no. 7 (2011).

110 Ibid.

111 L. H. Aiken et al., "Hospital Staffing, Organization, and Quality of Care: Cross-National Findings," Int J Qual Health Care 14, no. 1 (2002).

112 C. Dall'Ora et al., "Association of 12 H Shifts and Nurses' Job Satisfaction, Burnout and Intention to Leave: Findings from a Cross-Sectional Study of 12 European Countries," BMJ Open 5, no. 9 (2015).

113 R. J. Holden et al., "A Human Factors Framework and Study of the Effect of Nursing Workload on Patient Safety and Employee Quality of Working Life," BMJ Qual Saf 20, no. 1 (2011).

114 National Academies of Sciences.

115 E. G. Epstein et al., "Enhancing Understanding of Moral Distress: The Measure of Moral Distress for Health Care Professionals," AJOB Empir Bioeth 10, no. 2 (2019).

116 Ibid.; Rushton et al.

117 ; A. B. Hamric and L. J. Blackhall, "Nurse-Physician Perspectives on the Care of Dying Patients in Intensive Care Units: Collaboration, Moral Distress, and Ethical Climate," Crit Care Med 35, no. 2 (2007).

118 Rushton et al.

Chapter 8. The Stigma Surrounding Mental Health

119 R. Balon, "Psychiatrist Attitudes toward Self-Treatment of Their Own Depression," Psychother Psychosom 76, no. 5 (2007).

120 H. P. Grocott and G. L. Bryson, "The Physician at Risk: Disruptive Behaviour, Burnout, Addiction, and Suicide," Can J Anaesth 64, no. 2 (2017).

121 Luke 4:23-24 [NKJV]

122 M. C. Kalmoe et al., "Physician Suicide: A Call to Action," Mo Med 116, no. 3 (2019).

123 C. Center et al., "Confronting Depression and Suicide in Physicians: A Consensus Statement," JAMA 289, no. 23 (2003).

124 K. J. Gold et al., ""I Would Never Want to Have a Mental Health Diagnosis on My Record": A Survey of Female Physicians on Mental Health Diagnosis, Treatment, and Reporting," Gen Hosp Psychiatry 43 (2016).

125 J. T. R. Jones et al., "Medical Licensure Questions About Mental Illness and Compliance with the Americans with Disabilities Act," J Am Acad Psychiatry Law 46, no. 4 (2018).

126 R. Schroeder et al., "Do State Medical Board Applications Violate the Americans with Disabilities Act?," Acad Med 84, no. 6 (2009); Jones et al.

127 ADA National Network, "What Is the Americans with Disabilities Act (Ada)?," https://adata.org/learn-about-ada.

128 Jones et al.

129 American Psychiatric Association, "Position Statement on Confidentiality of Medical Records: Does the Physician Have a Right to Privacy Concerning His or Her Own Medical Records," Am J Psychiatry 141, no. 2 (1984).

130 Jones et al.

131 Center et al.

132 Jones et al.

133 Katherine J Gold et al., "Do Us Medical Licensing Applications Treat Mental and Physical Illness Equivalently?," Fam Med 49, no. 6 (2017).no. 6 (2017

134 American Psychiatric Association, "Position Statement on Inquiries About Diagnosis and Treatment of Mental Disordersin Connection with Professional Credentialing and Licensing," https://www.psychiatry.org/File%20 Library/About-APA/Organization-Documents-Policies/Policies/Position-2018-Inquiries-about-Diagnosis-and-Treatment-of-Mental-Disorders-in-Connection-with-Professional-Credentialing-and-Licensing.pdf; Federation of State Medical Boards, "Supplemental Resource: Report and Recommendations of the Fsmb Workgroup on Physician Wellness and Burnout," Journal of Medical Regulation 104, no. 2 (2018).

135 Kuhn and Flanagan.

136 M. J. Halter et al., "State Nursing Licensure Questions About Mental Illness and Compliance with the Americans with Disabilities Act," J Psychosoc Nurs Ment Health Serv 57, no. 8 (2019).

137 Maslach, "Finding Solutions to the Problem of Burnout."

138 D. G. Myers, "The Self in a Social World," in Social Psychology (New York: McGraw-Hill, 2012).

Chapter 9. Personality

139 K.L. Kumpfer, "Factors and Processes Contributing to Resilience: The Resilience Framework," in Resilience and Development: Positive Life Adapta-

tions, ed. M.D.; Johnson Glantz, J.L. (New York: Kluwer Academic Publishers, 1999).

140 C. S. Dweck, "Mindsets and Human Nature: Promoting Change in the Middle East, the Schoolyard, the Racial Divide, and Willpower," Am Psychol 67, no. 8 (2012).

141 Ibid.; Richard W. Robins and Jennifer L. Pals, "Implicit Self-Theories in the Academic Domain: Implications for Goal Orientation, Attributions, Affect, and Self-Esteem Change," Self and Identity 1, no. 4 (2002).

142 National Academies of Sciences.

143 Merriam-Webster, "Resilience".

144 C. P. West et al., "Resilience and Burnout among Physicians and the General Us Working Population," JAMA Netw Open 3, no. 7 (2020).

145 J. Brezo, J. Paris, and G. Turecki, "Personality Traits as Correlates of Suicidal Ideation, Suicide Attempts, and Suicide Completions: A Systematic Review," Acta Psychiatr Scand 113, no. 3 (2006).

146 Myers.

147 Kumpfer.

148 R. A. van der Wal et al., "Psychological Distress, Burnout and Personality Traits in Dutch Anaesthesiologists: A Survey," Eur J Anaesthesiol 33, no. 3 (2016); Y. Yao et al., "General Self-Efficacy Modifies the Effect of Stress on Burnout in Nurses with Different Personality Types," BMC Health Serv Res 18, no. 1 (2018).

149 M.R. Leary and R.H. Hoyle, Handbook of Individual Differences in Social Behavior (Guilford Publications, 2009).

150 Andrea P. Chioqueta and Tore C. Stiles, "Personality Traits and the Development of Depression, Hopelessness, and Suicide Ideation," Personality and Individual Differences 38, no. 6 (2005); M. W. Enns and B. J. Cox, "Personality Dimensions and Depression: Review and Commentary," Can J Psychiatry 42, no. 3 (1997); Drew M. Velting, "Suicidal Ideation and the Five-Factor Model of Personality," Personality and Individual Differences 27, no. 5 (1999); H. L. DeShong et al., "Five Factor Model Traits as a Predic-

tor of Suicide Ideation and Interpersonal Suicide Risk in a College Sample," Psychiatry Res 226, no. 1 (2015); M. Perrin et al., "Determinants of the Development of Post-Traumatic Stress Disorder, in the General Population," Soc Psychiatry Psychiatr Epidemiol 49, no. 3 (2014).

151 Andrew P. Hill and Thomas Curran, "Multidimensional Perfectionism and Burnout:A Meta-Analysis," Personality and Social Psychology Review 20, no. 3 (2016).

152 Gordon L. Flett and Paul L. Hewitt, "A Proposed Framework for Preventing Perfectionism and Promoting Resilience and Mental Health among Vulnerable Children and Adolescents " Psychology in the Schools 51, no. 9 (2014).

153 Ibid.

154 Reidar Tyssen, "Personality Traits," in Physician Mental Health and Well-Being: Research and Practice, ed. Kirk J. Brower and Michelle B. Riba (Cham: Springer International Publishing, 2017).

155 R. Tyssen, "Work and Mental Health in Doctors: A Short Review of Norwegian Studies," Porto Biomed J 4, no. 5 (2019).

156 K. Johnson, "Stressed Med Students at High Risk for Later Depression," Medscape, https://www.medscape.com/viewarticle/773650.

157 Myers.

158 D. J. Snowden and M. E. Boone, "A Leader's Framework for Decision Making. A Leader's Framework for Decision Making," Harv Bus Rev 85, no. 11 (2007).

159 J.; Gautam Van Aerde, M. , "Leadership Agility in Chaotic Systems," in Canadian Society of Physician Leaders Covid-19 Bulletin #2, ed. Canadian Society of Physician Leaders (Canadian Society of Physician Leaders, 2020).

160 Kuhn and Flanagan.

161 C. R. Stehman et al., "Burnout, Drop out, Suicide: Physician Loss in Emergency Medicine, Part I," West J Emerg Med 20, no. 3 (2019); A. W. Wu,

"Medical Error: The Second Victim. The Doctor Who Makes the Mistake Needs Help Too," BMJ 320, no. 7237 (2000).

162 Stehman et al.

163 L. A. Treiber and J. H. Jones, "Making an Infusion Error: The Second Victims of Infusion Therapy-Related Medication Errors," J Infus Nurs 41, no. 3 (2018); Zane Robinson Wolf et al., "Responses and Concerns of Healthcare Providers to Medication Errors," Clinical Nurse Specialist 14, no. 6 (2000).

164 Kuhn and Flanagan.

165 A. Nedrow, N. A. Steckler, and J. Hardman, "Physician Resilience and Burnout: Can You Make the Switch?," Fam Pract Manag 20, no. 1 (2013).

166 Kuhn and Flanagan.

167 Lisa Elliot, Jonathon Tan, and Sarah Norris, The Mental Health of Doctors: A Systematic Literature Review (Hawthorn West, Vic.: Beyondblue, 2010).

Chapter 10. Interventions and Coping Methods

168 G. A. Kenna and M. D. Wood, "Alcohol Use by Healthcare Professionals," Drug Alcohol Depend 75, no. 1 (2004).

169 C. Maslach, Jackson, S.E., and Leiter, M.P., Maslach Burnout Inventory, 3 ed. (Palo Alto, California: Consulting Psychologists Press, 1996).

170 National Academies of Sciences.

171 Maslach and Leiter.

172 Maslach.

173 P. Koutsimani, A. Montgomery, and K. Georganta, "The Relationship between Burnout, Depression, and Anxiety: A Systematic Review and Meta-Analysis," Front Psychol 10 (2019); Maslach and Leiter.

174 M. Myers and C. Fine, "Suicide in Physicians: Toward Prevention," MedGenMed 5, no. 4 (2003).

175 Louise B. Andrew, "Physician Suicide," https://emedicine.medscape.com/article/806779-overview#a5.

176 Douglas A. Sargent et al., "Preventing Physician Suicide: The Role of Family, Colleagues, and Organized Medicine," JAMA 237, no. 2 (1977); M. Ross, "Suicide among Physicians," Psychiatry Med 2, no. 3 (1971).

177 Andrew.

178 American Association of Suicidology, "Warning Signs," http://suicidology.org/resources/warning-signs/.

179 J. D. Yoon et al., "Physician Burnout and the Calling to Care for the Dying: A National Survey," Am J Hosp Palliat Care 34, no. 10 (2017).

180 Ibid.

181 S. Folkman and R. S. Lazarus, "An Analysis of Coping in a Middle-Aged Community Sample," J Health Soc Behav 21, no. 3 (1980).

182 Hyojung Shin et al., "Relationships between Coping Strategies and Burnout Symptoms: A Meta-Analytic Approach," Professional Psychology: Research and Practice 45 (2014).

183 C. S. Carver, M. F. Scheier, and J. K. Weintraub, "Assessing Coping Strategies: A Theoretically Based Approach," J Pers Soc Psychol 56, no. 2 (1989).

184 C. Maslach, W. B. Schaufeli, and M. P. Leiter, "Job Burnout," Annu Rev Psychol 52 (2001).

185 Shin et al.

186 Ibid.

187 A. Chiesa and P. Malinowski, "Mindfulness-Based Approaches: Are They All the Same?," J Clin Psychol 67, no. 4 (2011).

188 Ibid.

189 Ibid.

190 M. Goyal et al., "Meditation Programs for Psychological Stress and Well-Being: A Systematic Review and Meta-Analysis," JAMA Intern Med 174, no. 3 (2014).

191 S. A. Kriakous et al., "The Effectiveness of Mindfulness-Based Stress Reduction on the Psychological Functioning of Healthcare Professionals: A Systematic Review," Mindfulness (N Y) (2020); Brittany F. Escuriex and Elise E. Labbé, "Health Care Providers' Mindfulness and Treatment Outcomes:

A Critical Review of the Research Literature," Mindfulness 2, no. 4 (2011); Colin P. West et al., "Interventions to Prevent and Reduce Physician Burnout: A Systematic Review and Meta-Analysis," The Lancet 388, no. 10057 (2016).

192 Panagioti et al.

193 Ibid.

194 West et al.

195 L. N. Dyrbye et al., "Effect of a Professional Coaching Intervention on the Well-Being and Distress of Physicians: A Pilot Randomized Clinical Trial," JAMA Intern Med 179, no. 10 (2019).

Chapter 11. Debt and Financial Burdens

196 West, Shanafelt, and Kolars; Wisenberg Brin.

197 A. Bazemore et al., "Over Half of Graduating Family Medicine Residents Report More Than $150,000 in Educational Debt," J Am Board Fam Med 29, no. 2 (2016); J. Phillips, "The Impact of Debt on Young Family Physicians: Unanswered Questions with Critical Implications," ibid.

198 M. S. Grayson, D. A. Newton, and L. F. Thompson, "Payback Time: The Associations of Debt and Income with Medical Student Career Choice," Med Educ 46, no. 10 (2012).

199 Wisenberg Brin.

200 Benjamin T. B. Chan, "From Perceived Surplus to Perceived Shortage: What Happened to Canadaís Physician Workforce in the 1990s?," (2002), https://secure.cihi.ca/free_products/chanjun02.pdf.

201 Ibid.

202 National Resident Matching Program, "Advance Data Tables 2021 Main Residency Match," https://mk0nrmp3oyqui6wqfm.kinstacdn.com/wp-content/uploads/2021/03/Advance-Data-Tables-2021_Final.pdf.

203 Canadian Resident Matching Service, "Table 1: Summary of Match Results," https://www.carms.ca/wp-content/uploads/2021/06/r1_tbl1e.pdf; "2021 Carms Forum," https://carms.ca/pdfs/2021-carms-forum.pdf.

204 "Table 3: Summary of Positions by School of Residency," https://www.carms.ca/wp-content/uploads/2020/05/2020_r1_tbl3e.pdf.

205 "Table 1: Summary of Match Results," https://www.carms.ca/wp-content/uploads/2020/05/2020_r1_tbl1e.pdf.

206 National Resident Matching Program, "Charting Outcomes in the Match: International Medical Graduates," https://mk0nrmp3oyqui6wqfm.kinstacdn.com/wp-content/uploads/2020/07/Charting-Outcomes-in-the-Match-2020_IMG_final.pdf.

207 American Society of Physicians, "Support for Assistant Physician Licenses," https://www.linkedin.com/posts/asphysicians_ap-license-support-statement-activity-6703677529443631104-DCl-.

208 Ibid.

209 M. P. Salyers et al., "The Relationship between Professional Burnout and Quality and Safety in Healthcare: A Meta-Analysis," J Gen Intern Med 32, no. 4 (2017); C. S. Dewa et al., "The Relationship between Physician Burnout and Quality of Healthcare in Terms of Safety and Acceptability: A Systematic Review," BMJ Open 7, no. 6 (2017).

Chapter 12. Medical Errors

210 D. S. Tawfik et al., "Physician Burnout, Well-Being, and Work Unit Safety Grades in Relationship to Reported Medical Errors," Mayo Clin Proc 93, no. 11 (2018); N. K. Menon et al., "Association of Physician Burnout with Suicidal Ideation and Medical Errors," JAMA Netw Open 3, no. 12 (2020); E. K. Kang, H. S. Lihm, and E. H. Kong, "Association of Intern and Resident Burnout with Self-Reported Medical Errors," Korean J Fam Med 34, no. 1 (2013).

211 Tawfik et al.

212 L. N.; Shanafelt Dyrbye, T. D.; Sinsky, C. A.; Cipriano, P. F.; Bhatt J.; Ommaya, A.; West, C. P.; Meyers, D., "Burnout among Health Care Professionals: A Call to Explore and Address This Underrecognized Threat to Safe, High-Quality Care," National Academy of Medicine, https://nam.edu/

burnout-among-health-care-professionals-a-call-to-explore-and-address-this-underrecognized-threat-to-safe-high-quality-care/.

213 A. K. Windover et al., "Correlates and Outcomes of Physician Burnout within a Large Academic Medical Center," JAMA Intern Med 178, no. 6 (2018).

214 Salyers et al.

215 Ibid.; Michael P. Leiter, Phyllis Harvie, and Cindy Frizzell, "The Correspondence of Patient Satisfaction and Nurse Burnout," Social Science & Medicine 47, no. 10 (1998); R. G. Carey and J. H. Seibert, "A Patient Survey System to Measure Quality Improvement: Questionnaire Reliability and Validity," Med Care 31, no. 9 (1993).

216 E. M. White, L. H. Aiken, and M. D. McHugh, "Registered Nurse Burnout, Job Dissatisfaction, and Missed Care in Nursing Homes," J Am Geriatr Soc 67, no. 10 (2019).

217 L. Donaldson, "An Organisation with a Memory," Clin Med (Lond) 2, no. 5 (2002).

218 Medicine Institute of, To Err Is Human: Building a Safer Health System, ed. T. Kohn Linda, M. Corrigan Janet, and S. Donaldson Molla (Washington, DC: The National Academies Press, 2000).

219 Ibid.; J. Reason, Managing the Risks of Organizational Accidents (Routledge, 2016).

220 Institute of.

221 APA Dictionary of Psychology, "Hindsight Bias," American Psychology Association, https://dictionary.apa.org/hindsight-bias.

222 Federal Aviation Administration, "Flightcrew Member Duty and Rest Requirements," https://www.faa.gov/regulations_policies/rulemaking/recently_published/media/2120-AJ58-FinalRule.pdf.

Chapter 13. Exhaustion

223 Ibid.

224 S. Banks and D. F. Dinges, "Behavioral and Physiological Consequences of Sleep Restriction," J Clin Sleep Med 3, no. 5 (2007); H. P. Van Dongen et al., "The Cumulative Cost of Additional Wakefulness: Dose-Response Effects on Neurobehavioral Functions and Sleep Physiology from Chronic Sleep Restriction and Total Sleep Deprivation," Sleep 26, no. 2 (2003).

225 Van Dongen et al.

226 G. Belenky et al., "Patterns of Performance Degradation and Restoration During Sleep Restriction and Subsequent Recovery: A Sleep Dose-Response Study," J Sleep Res 12, no. 1 (2003).

227 Ibid.

228 A. M. Williamson and A. M. Feyer, "Moderate Sleep Deprivation Produces Impairments in Cognitive and Motor Performance Equivalent to Legally Prescribed Levels of Alcohol Intoxication," Occup Environ Med 57, no. 10 (2000).

229 Paul Maruff et al., "Fatigue-Related Impairment in the Speed, Accuracy and Variability of Psychomotor Performance: Comparison with Blood Alcohol Levels," Journal of Sleep Research 14, no. 1 (2005).

230 Matthew Walker, Why We Sleep (Harlow, England: Penguin Books, 2018).

231 Laura K. Barger et al., "Extended Work Shifts and the Risk of Motor Vehicle Crashes among Interns," New England Journal of Medicine 352, no. 2 (2005).

232 M. Basner et al., "Sleep and Alertness in Medical Interns and Residents: An Observational Study on the Role of Extended Shifts," Sleep 40, no. 4 (2017).

233 J. A. Shea et al., "A Randomized Trial of a Three-Hour Protected Nap Period in a Medicine Training Program: Sleep, Alertness, and Patient Outcomes," Acad Med 89, no. 3 (2014).

234 Kuhn and Flanagan.

235 Ibid.

236 Pulse, "Number of Registered Patients Per Gp Rises to Almost 2,100," https://www.pulsetoday.co.uk/news/workload/number-of-registered-pa-

tients-per-gp-rises-to-almost-2100/; B. White and D. Twiddy, "The State of Family Medicine: 2017," Fam Pract Manag 24, no. 1 (2017).

Chapter 14. Mental (Un)Wellness

237 Centre.

238 K. Ahola et al., "Burnout as a Predictor of All-Cause Mortality among Industrial Employees: A 10-Year Prospective Register-Linkage Study," J Psychosom Res 69, no. 1 (2010).

239 Maslach; National Academies of Sciences.

240 T. D. Shanafelt et al., "Special Report: Suicidal Ideation among American Surgeons," Arch Surg 146, no. 1 (2011).

241 Ibid.; F. van der Heijden et al., "Suicidal Thoughts among Medical Residents with Burnout," Arch Suicide Res 12, no. 4 (2008); L. N. Dyrbye et al., "Burnout and Suicidal Ideation among U.S. Medical Students," Ann Intern Med 149, no. 5 (2008).

242 Menon et al.

243 Association.

244 T. D. Shanafelt et al., "Suicidal Ideation and Attitudes Regarding Help Seeking in Us Physicians Relative to the Us Working Population," Mayo Clin Proc 96, no. 8 (2021).

245 A. M. Stelnicki et al., "Suicidal Behaviors among Nurses in Canada," Can J Nurs Res 52, no. 3 (2020).

246 A. Fridner et al., "Survey on Recent Suicidal Ideation among Female University Hospital Physicians in Sweden and Italy (the Houpe Study): Cross-Sectional Associations with Work Stressors," Gend Med 6, no. 1 (2009).

247 A. Fridner et al., "Work Environment and Recent Suicidal Thoughts among Male University Hospital Physicians in Sweden and Italy: The Health and Organization among University Hospital Physicians in Europe (Houpe) Study," ibid.8, no. 4 (2011).

248 M. Dong et al., "Prevalence of Suicide-Related Behaviors among Physicians: A Systematic Review and Meta-Analysis," Suicide Life Threat Behav 50, no. 6 (2020).

249 E. Bailey, J. Robinson, and P. McGorry, "Depression and Suicide among Medical Practitioners in Australia," Intern Med J 48, no. 3 (2018).

250 S. Sen et al., "A Prospective Cohort Study Investigating Factors Associated with Depression During Medical Internship," Arch Gen Psychiatry 67, no. 6 (2010).

251 Kalmoe et al; K. J. Gold, A. Sen, and T. L. Schwenk, "Details on Suicide among Us Physicians: Data from the National Violent Death Reporting System," Gen Hosp Psychiatry 35, no. 1 (2013).

252 Dyrbye; Yanhong Gong et al., "Prevalence of Depressive Symptoms and Work-Related Risk Factors among Nurses in Public Hospitals in Southern China: A Cross-Sectional Study," Scientific Reports 4, no. 1 (2014); S. Letvak, C. J. Ruhm, and T. McCoy, "Depression in Hospital-Employed Nurses," Clin Nurse Spec 26, no. 3 (2012); D. Welsh, "Predictors of Depressive Symptoms in Female Medical-Surgical Hospital Nurses," Issues Ment Health Nurs 30, no. 5 (2009); M. C. Ohler, M. S. Kerr, and D. A. Forbes, "Depression in Nurses," Can J Nurs Res 42, no. 3 (2010).

253 National Institute of Mental Health, "Major Depression," https://www. nimh.nih.gov/health/statistics/major-depression.

254 World Health Organization, "Depression," https://www.who.int/newsroom/fact-sheets/detail/depression.

255 V. J. Sutherland and C. L. Cooper, "Identifying Distress among General Practitioners: Predictors of Psychological Ill-Health and Job Dissatisfaction," Social Science & Medicine 37, no. 5 (1993).

256 D. A. Mata et al., "Prevalence of Depression and Depressive Symptoms among Resident Physicians: A Systematic Review and Meta-Analysis," JAMA 314, no. 22 (2015).

257 L. S. Rotenstein et al., "Prevalence of Depression, Depressive Symptoms, and Suicidal Ideation among Medical Students: A Systematic Review and Meta-Analysis," ibid.316, no. 21 (2016).

258 D. A. Mata et al., "Prevalence of Depression and Depressive Symptoms among Resident Physicians: A Systematic Review and Meta-Analysis," ibid.314, no. 22 (2015).

259 A. M. Shangraw et al., "Prevalence of Anxiety and Depressive Symptoms among Pharmacy Students," Am J Pharm Educ 85, no. 2 (2021).

260 Y. J. Tung et al., "Prevalence of Depression among Nursing Students: A Systematic Review and Meta-Analysis," Nurse Educ Today 63 (2018).

261 Bailey, Robinson, and McGorry.

262 Shanafelt et al.

263 Jane L. Givens and Jennifer Tjia, "Depressed Medical Students' Use of Mental Health Services and Barriers to Use," Academic Medicine 77, no. 9 (2002).

264 C. M. Brazeau et al., "Distress among Matriculating Medical Students Relative to the General Population," Acad Med 89, no. 11 (2014).

265 Tung et al.

266 Andrew.

267 Elliot, Tan, and Norris.

268 K. Hawton et al., "Suicide in Doctors: A Study of Risk According to Gender, Seniority and Specialty in Medical Practitioners in England and Wales, 1979-1995," J Epidemiol Community Health 55, no. 5 (2001); S. Lindeman et al., "A Systematic Review on Gender-Specific Suicide Mortality in Medical Doctors," Br J Psychiatry 168, no. 3 (1996).

269 Kalmoe et al.

270 Ibid.

271 T. D. Shanafelt et al., «Changes in Burnout and Satisfaction with Work-Life Integration in Physicians and the General Us Working Population between 2011 and 2017,» Mayo Clin Proc 94, no. 9 (2019).

272 C. Peterson et al., "Suicide Rates by Major Occupational Group - 17 States, 2012 and 2015," MMWR Morb Mortal Wkly Rep 67, no. 45 (2018).

273 Carpenter, Swerdlow, and Fear; Ko et al.

274 C. W. Drapeau, McIntosh, J. L. (for the American and Association of Suicidology), "U.S.A. Suicide: 2018 Official Final Data," American Association of Suicidology, http://www.suicidology.org; N. A. Yaghmour et al., "Causes of Death of Residents in Acgme-Accredited Programs 2000 through 2014: Implications for the Learning Environment," Acad Med 92, no. 7 (2017).

275 Erica Frank, Holly Biola, and Carol A. Burnett, "Mortality Rates and Causes among U.S. Physicians," American Journal of Preventive Medicine 19, no. 3 (2000).

276 National Academies of Sciences; Shanafelt et al; C. M. Balch et al., "Distress and Career Satisfaction among 14 Surgical Specialties, Comparing Academic and Private Practice Settings," Ann Surg 254, no. 4 (2011).

277 F. Dutheil et al., "Suicide among Physicians and Health-Care Workers: A Systematic Review and Meta-Analysis," PLoS One 14, no. 12 (2019).

278 Kuhn and Flanagan.

279 Association.

280 Sargent et al.

281 L. G. Lefebvre and I. M. Kaufmann, "The Identification and Management of Substance Use Disorders in Anesthesiologists," Can J Anaesth 64, no. 2 (2017); M. R. Oreskovich et al., "The Prevalence of Substance Use Disorders in American Physicians," Am J Addict 24, no. 1 (2015).

282 Physician Health Monitoring Committee, "Substance Use and Behavioural Disorders Definitions," College of Physicians & Surgeons of Alberta, http://www.cpsa.ca/physician-health-monitoring-program-phmp/phmp-policies/definitions/#:~:text=Canadian%20Society%20of%20Addiction%20Medicine,psychological%2C%20social%20and%20spiritual%20manifestations.

283 A. T. McLellan et al., "Five Year Outcomes in a Cohort Study of Physicians Treated for Substance Use Disorders in the United States," BMJ 337 (2008).

284 Gregory E. Skipper, Michael D. Campbell, and Robert L. DuPont, "Anesthesiologists with Substance Use Disorders: A 5-Year Outcome Study from 16 State Physician Health Programs," Anesthesia & Analgesia 109, no. 3 (2009).

285 Oreskovich et al.

286 Substance Abuse and Mental Health Services Administration, "Key Substance Use and Mental Health Indicators in the United States: Results from the 2018 National Survey on Drug Use and Health," Department of Health and Human Services (HHS), https://www.samhsa.gov/data/sites/default/files/cbhsq-reports/NSDUHNationalFindingsReport2018/NSDUHNationalFindingsReport2018.pdf.

287 Lefebvre and Kaufmann; E. O. Bryson and J. H. Silverstein, "Addiction and Substance Abuse in Anesthesiology," Anesthesiology 109, no. 5 (2008).

288 Lefebvre and Kaufmann.

289 Ibid.

290 J. M. Brewster et al., "Characteristics and Outcomes of Doctors in a Substance Dependence Monitoring Programme in Canada: Prospective Descriptive Study," BMJ 337 (2008).

291 Dyrbye.

292 Association.

293 National Academies of Sciences; Shanafelt et al.

294 M. Linzer and E. Harwood, "Gendered Expectations: Do They Contribute to High Burnout among Female Physicians?," J Gen Intern Med 33, no. 6 (2018).

295 Ibid.

296 M. Schmid Mast, J. A. Hall, and D. L. Roter, "Disentangling Physician Sex and Physician Communication Style: Their Effects on Patient Satisfaction in a Virtual Medical Visit," Patient Educ Couns 68, no. 1 (2007).

297 G. Cousin, M. Schmid Mast, and N. Jaunin-Stalder, "When Physician-Expressed Uncertainty Leads to Patient Dissatisfaction: A Gender Study," Med Educ 47, no. 9 (2013).

298 J. E. McMurray et al., "The Work Lives of Women Physicians Results from the Physician Work Life Study. The Sgim Career Satisfaction Study Group," Journal of general internal medicine 15, no. 6 (2000).

299 Ibid.; A. B. Jena, A. R. Olenski, and D. M. Blumenthal, "Sex Differences in Physician Salary in Us Public Medical Schools," JAMA Intern Med 176, no. 9 (2016).

300 Jena et al.

301 V.M.; Lautenberger Dandar, D.M., "Exploring Faculty Salary Equity at U.S. Medical Schools by Gender and Race/Ethnicity," (Washington, D.C.: Association of American Medical Colleges, 2021)." (Washington, D.C.: Association of American Medical Colleges, 2021

302 McMurray et al.

303 Panagioti et al.

304 T. Shanafelt, J. Ripp, and M. Trockel, "Understanding and Addressing Sources of Anxiety among Health Care Professionals During the Covid-19 Pandemic," JAMA 323, no. 21 (2020).

305 Ibid.

306 N. Khan et al., "Cross-Sectional Survey on Physician Burnout During the Covid-19 Pandemic in Vancouver, Canada: The Role of Gender, Ethnicity and Sexual Orientation," BMJ Open 11, no. 5 (2021).

307 Yi Quan Tan et al., "Psychological Health of Surgeons in a Time of Covid-19: A Global Survey," Annals of Surgery (2021).

308 Khan et al.

Chapter 15. Medical Errors and Disengaged Personnel

309 World Health Organization, "10 Facts on Patient Safety," https://www.who.int/news-room/photo-story/photo-story-detail/10-facts-on-patient-safety.

310 Lucian L. Leape, "Medical Errors and Patient Safety," in The Trust Crisis in Healthcare: Causes, Consequences, and Cures, ed. David A. Shore (New York: Oxford University Press, 2007).Consequences, and Cures</style>, ed. David A. Shore (New York: Oxford University Press, 2007

311 Martin A. Makary and Michael Daniel, "Medical Error—the Third Leading Cause of Death in the Us," BMJ 353 (2016).

312 World Health Organization, "International Classification of Diseases (Icd) Revision," https://www.who.int/classifications/icd/revision/icd11faq/en/.

313 Makary and Daniel.

314 Ibid.

315 World Health Organization, "Icd-11 for Mortality and Morbidity Statistics," https://icd.who.int/browse11/l-m/en#/http://id.who.int/icd/entity/129180281.

316 Institute of.

317 World Health Organization, "The Conceptual Framework for the International Classification for Patient Safety," https://www.who.int/publications/i/item/the-conceptual-framework-for-the-international-classification-for-patient-safety-(icps).

318 Institute of.

319 Ibid.; Makary and Daniel.

320 Kaveh G. Shojania and Mary Dixon-Woods, "Estimating Deaths Due to Medical Error: The Ongoing Controversy and Why It Matters," BMJ Quality & Safety 26, no. 5 (2017).

321 B.; Cochrane Chan, D., Measuring Patient Harm in Canadian Hospitals. With What Can Be Done to Improve Patient Safety?, (Ottawa, ON: Canadian Institute for Health Information, Canadian Patient Safety Institute., 2016).

322 Statistics Canada, "Table 13-10-0394-01 Leading Causes of Death, Total Population, by Age Group," Statistics Canada, https://www150.statcan.gc.ca/t1/tbl1/en/tv.action?pid=1310039401; RiskAnalytica, "The Case for Investing in Patient Safety in Canada," (2017), https://www.patientsafetyinstitute.ca/en/toolsResources/Documents/Patient%20Harm%20Awareness%20-%20Ipsos/Risk%20Analytica%202017%20The%20Case%20for%20Investing%20in%20Patient%20Safety%20in%20Canada.pdf.

323 Donaldson.

324 Hourse of Commons Health Committee, "Sixth Report Patient Safe-ty," https://publications.parliament.uk/pa/cm200809/cmselect/cm-health/151/15106.htm#a2.

325 R. M. Wilson et al., "The Quality in Australian Health Care Study," Med J Aust 163, no. 9 (1995).

326 Ibid.; Donaldson.

327 Organization, "10 Facts on Patient Safety"; Luke Slawomirski, Ane Au-raaen, and Niek S. Klazinga, "The Economics of Patient Safety: Strengthen-ing a Value-Based Approach to Reducing Patient Harm at National Level" (paper presented at the 2nd Global Ministerial Summit on Patient Safety, Bonn, Germany, 2017).

328 Shojania and Dixon-Woods.

329 World Health Organization, "Reporting and Learning Systems," https://www.who.int/patientsafety/topics/reporting-learning/en/.

Chapter 16. Understanding the Costs of Burnout

330 National Academies of Sciences.

331 L. H. Aiken et al., "Patient Safety, Satisfaction, and Quality of Hospital Care: Cross Sectional Surveys of Nurses and Patients in 12 Countries in Europe and the United States," BMJ 344 (2012).

332 J. R. Halbesleben and C. Rathert, "Linking Physician Burnout and Patient Outcomes: Exploring the Dyadic Relationship between Physicians and Pa-tients," Health Care Manage Rev 33, no. 1 (2008); Dyrbye.

333 C. A. Sinsky et al., "Professional Satisfaction and the Career Plans of Us Physicians," Mayo Clin Proc 92, no. 11 (2017); National Academies of Sci-ences.

334 S. Han et al., "Estimating the Attributable Cost of Physician Burnout in the United States," Ann Intern Med 170, no. 11 (2019).

335 C. S. Dewa et al., "An Estimate of the Cost of Burnout on Early Retirement and Reduction in Clinical Hours of Practicing Physicians in Canada," BMC Health Serv Res 14 (2014).

336 C. B. Jones, "The Costs of Nurse Turnover, Part 2: Application of the Nursing Turnover Cost Calculation Methodology," J Nurs Adm 35, no. 1 (2005); "Revisiting Nurse Turnover Costs: Adjusting for Inflation," J Nurs Adm 38, no. 1 (2008); Dyrbye.

337 World Health Organization, "Icd-10 Version:2019," https://icd.who.int/browse10/2019/en#/Z73.

338 "Icd-11 for Mortality and Morbidity Statistics".

339 Ibid.

340 W.B. Schaufeli, M.P. Leiter, and C. Maslach, "Burnout: 35 Years of Research and Practice," Career Development International 14, no. 3 (2009).

341 Maslach and Leiter.

342 Ibid.

343 Schaufeli, Leiter, and Maslach.

344 A. Lastovkova et al., "Burnout Syndrome as an Occupational Disease in the European Union: An Exploratory Study," Ind Health 56, no. 2 (2018).

345 Maslach and Leiter.

346 Ibid.

347 S. T. Gregory, T. Menser, and B. T. Gregory, „An Organizational Intervention to Reduce Physician Burnout," J Healthc Manag 63, no. 5 (2018).

348 P. M. Dunn et al., "Meeting the Imperative to Improve Physician Well-Being: Assessment of an Innovative Program," J Gen Intern Med 22, no. 11 (2007).

349 Ibid.

350 R. J. Reid et al., "The Group Health Medical Home at Year Two: Cost Savings, Higher Patient Satisfaction, and Less Burnout for Providers," Health Aff (Millwood) 29, no. 5 (2010).

351 Ibid.

Chapter 17. The Cost of Adverse Events

352 RiskAnalytica.

353 Chan.

354 Slawomirski, Auraaen, and Klazinga.

355 Ibid.

356 K. D. Hauck et al., "Healthy Life-Years Lost and Excess Bed-Days Due to 6 Patient Safety Incidents: Empirical Evidence from English Hospitals," Med Care 55, no. 2 (2017).

357 Chan.

358 Hauck et al.

359 Slawomirski, Auraaen, and Klazinga.

360 Ibid.

361 Ibid.

362 C. E. Mahan et al., "Deep-Vein Thrombosis: A United States Cost Model for a Preventable and Costly Adverse Event," Thromb Haemost 106, no. 3 (2011).

363 Ibid.; Slawomirski, Auraaen, and Klazinga.

Chapter 18. Six Strategies to Address Burnout

364 Pascale Carayon, Christine Cassel, and Victor J. Dzau, "Improving the System to Support Clinician Well-Being and Provide Better Patient Care," JAMA 322, no. 22 (2019); National Academies of Sciences.

REFERENCES

(NIOSH), National Institute for Occupational Safety and Health. "Occupational Health Safety Network (OHSN)." Centers for Disease Control and Prevention. Last modified September 30, 2019. https://www.cdc.gov/niosh/topics/ohsn/.

———. "Occupational Violence Fast Facts." Centers for Disease Control and Prevention. Last modified September 22, 2020. https://www.cdc.gov/niosh/topics/violence/fastfacts.html.

Acquadro Maran, D., C. G. Cortese, P. Pavanelli, G. Fornero, and M. M. Gianino. "Gender Differences in Reporting Workplace Violence: A Qualitative Analysis of Administrative Records of Violent Episodes Experienced by Healthcare Workers in a Large Public Italian Hospital." *BMJ Open* 9, no. 11 (Nov 10 2019): e031546.

Administration, Federal Aviation. "Flightcrew Member Duty and Rest Requirements." Accessed June 14, 2020. https://www.faa.gov/regulations_policies/rulemaking/recently_published/media/2120-AJ58-FinalRule.pdf.

Administration, Substance Abuse and Mental Health Services. "Key Substance Use and Mental Health Indicators in the United States: Results from the 2018 National Survey on Drug Use and Health." Department of Health and Human Services (HHS). Accessed October 5, 2020. https://www.samhsa.gov/data/sites/default/files/cbhsq-reports/NSDUHNationalFindingsReport2018/NSDUHNationalFindingsReport2018.pdf.

Ahola, K., A. Vaananen, A. Koskinen, A. Kouvonen, and A. Shirom. "Burnout as a Predictor of All-Cause Mortality among Industrial Employees: A 10-Year Prospective Register-Linkage Study." *J Psychosom Res* 69, no. 1 (Jul 2010): 51-7.

Aiken, L. H., S. P. Clarke, D. M. Sloane, and Consortium International Hospital Outcomes Research. "Hospital Staffing, Organization, and Quality of Care: Cross-National Findings." *Int J Qual Health Care* 14, no. 1 (Feb 2002): 5-13.

Aiken, L. H., W. Sermeus, K. Van den Heede, D. M. Sloane, R. Busse, M. McKee, L. Bruyneel, *et al.* "Patient Safety, Satisfaction, and Quality of Hospital Care: Cross Sectional Surveys of Nurses and Patients in 12 Countries in Europe and the United States." *BMJ* 344 (Mar 20 2012): e1717.

Ali, N. A., J. Hammersley, S. P. Hoffmann, J. M. O'Brien, Jr., G. S. Phillips, M. Rashkin, E. Warren, A. Garland, and Consortium Midwest Critical Care. "Continuity of Care in Intensive Care Units: A Cluster-Randomized Trial of Intensivist Staffing." *Am J Respir Crit Care Med* 184, no. 7 (Oct 1 2011): 803-8.

Andrew, Louise B. "Physician Suicide." Last modified August 1, 2018. https://emedicine.medscape.com/article/806779-overview#a5.

Arndt, B. G., J. W. Beasley, M. D. Watkinson, J. L. Temte, W. J. Tuan, C. A. Sinsky, and V. J. Gilchrist. "Tethered to the Ehr: Primary Care Physician Workload Assessment Using Ehr Event Log Data and Time-Motion Observations." *Ann Fam Med* 15, no. 5 (Sep 2017): 419-26.

Association, American Psychiatric. "Position Statement on Confidentiality of Medical Records: Does the Physician Have a Right to Privacy Concerning His or Her Own Medical Records." *Am J Psychiatry* 141, no. 2 (1984): 331-32.

———. "Position Statement on Inquiries About Diagnosis and Treatment of Mental Disorders in Connection with Professional Credentialing and Licensing." Accessed September 1, 2021. https://www.psychiatry.org/File%20Library/About-APA/Organization-Documents-Policies/Policies/Position-2018-Inquiries-about-Diagnosis-and-Treatment-of-Mental-Disorders-in-Connection-with-Professional-Credentialing-and-Licensing.pdf.

Association, Canadian Medical. "Cma National Physician Health Survey." Canadian Medical Association. Accessed June 27, 2020. https://www.cma.ca/sites/default/files/2018-11/nph-survey-e.pdf.

Bailey, E., J. Robinson, and P. McGorry. "Depression and Suicide among Medical Practitioners in Australia." *Intern Med J* 48, no. 3 (Mar 2018): 254-58.

Bakker Arnold, B., and Evangelia Demerouti. "The Job Demands-Resources Model: State of the Art." *Journal of Managerial Psychology* 22, no. 3 (2007): 309-28.

Balch, C. M., T. D. Shanafelt, J. A. Sloan, D. V. Satele, and J. A. Freischlag. "Distress and Career Satisfaction among 14 Surgical Specialties, Comparing Academic and Private Practice Settings." *Ann Surg* 254, no. 4 (Oct 2011): 558-68.

Balon, R. "Psychiatrist Attitudes toward Self-Treatment of Their Own Depression." *Psychother Psychosom* 76, no. 5 (2007): 306-10.

Banks, S., and D. F. Dinges. "Behavioral and Physiological Consequences of Sleep Restriction." *J Clin Sleep Med* 3, no. 5 (Aug 15 2007): 519-28.

Barger, Laura K., Brian E. Cade, Najib T. Ayas, John W. Cronin, Bernard Rosner, Frank E. Speizer, and Charles A. Czeisler. "Extended Work Shifts and the Risk of Motor Vehicle Crashes among Interns." *New England Journal of Medicine* 352, no. 2 (2005): 125-34.

Basner, M., D. F. Dinges, J. A. Shea, D. S. Small, J. Zhu, L. Norton, A. J. Ecker, *et al.* "Sleep and Alertness in Medical Interns and Residents: An Observational Study on the Role of Extended Shifts." *Sleep* 40, no. 4 (Apr 1 2017).

Bazemore, A., L. Peterson, A. Jetty, P. Wingrove, S. Petterson, and R. Phillips. "Over Half of Graduating Family Medicine Residents Report More Than $150,000 in Educational Debt." *J Am Board Fam Med* 29, no. 2 (Mar-Apr 2016): 180-1.

Belenky, G., N. J. Wesensten, D. R. Thorne, M. L. Thomas, H. C. Sing, D. P. Redmond, M. B. Russo, and T. J. Balkin. "Patterns of Performance Degradation and Restoration During Sleep Restriction and Subsequent Recovery: A Sleep Dose-Response Study." *J Sleep Res* 12, no. 1 (Mar 2003): 1-12.

Berwick, D. M., T. W. Nolan, and J. Whittington. "The Triple Aim: Care, Health, and Cost." *Health Aff (Millwood)* 27, no. 3 (May-Jun 2008): 759-69.

Block, L., R. Habicht, A. W. Wu, S. V. Desai, K. Wang, K. N. Silva, T. Niessen, N. Oliver, and L. Feldman. "In the Wake of the 2003 and 2011 Duty Hours Regulations, How Do Internal Medicine Interns Spend Their Time?". *J Gen Intern Med* 28, no. 8 (Aug 2013): 1042-7.

Boards, Federation of State Medical. "Supplemental Resource: Report and Recommendations of the Fsmb Workgroup on Physician Wellness and Burnout." *Journal of Medical Regulation* 104, no. 2 (2018): 37-48.

Bodenheimer, T., and C. Sinsky. "From Triple to Quadruple Aim: Care of the Patient Requires Care of the Provider." *Ann Fam Med* 12, no. 6 (Nov-Dec 2014): 573-6.

Brazeau, C. M., T. Shanafelt, S. J. Durning, F. S. Massie, A. Eacker, C. Moutier, D. V. Satele, J. A. Sloan, and L. N. Dyrbye. "Distress among Matriculating Medical Students Relative to the General Population." *Acad Med* 89, no. 11 (Nov 2014): 1520-5.

Brewster, J. M., I. M. Kaufmann, S. Hutchison, and C. MacWilliam. "Characteristics and Outcomes of Doctors in a Substance Dependence Monitoring Programme in Canada: Prospective Descriptive Study." *BMJ* 337 (Nov 3 2008): a2098.

Brezo, J., J. Paris, and G. Turecki. "Personality Traits as Correlates of Suicidal Ideation, Suicide Attempts, and Suicide Completions: A Systematic Review." *Acta Psychiatr Scand* 113, no. 3 (Mar 2006): 180-206.

Brough, Paula. "Workplace Violence Experienced by Paramedics: Relationships with Social Support, Job Satisfaction, and Psychological Strain." *Australas. J. Disast. Trauma Stud.* 2 (01/01 2005).

Bryson, E. O., and J. H. Silverstein. "Addiction and Substance Abuse in Anesthesiology." *Anesthesiology* 109, no. 5 (Nov 2008): 905-17.

Burgoon, J.K., L.K. Guerrero, and V. Manusov. *Nonverbal Communication*. Routledge, 2016.

Canada, Statistics. "Table 13-10-0394-01 Leading Causes of Death, Total Population, by Age Group." Statistics Canada. Last modified November 7, 2021. https://www150.statcan.gc.ca/t1/tbl1/en/tv.action?pid=1310039401.

Carayon, Pascale. "The Balance Theory and the Work System Model ... Twenty Years Later." *International Journal of Human-Computer Interaction* 25, no. 5 (2009): 313-27.

Carayon, Pascale, Christine Cassel, and Victor J. Dzau. "Improving the System to Support Clinician Well-Being and Provide Better Patient Care." *JAMA* 322, no. 22 (2019): 2165-66.

Carey, R. G., and J. H. Seibert. "A Patient Survey System to Measure Quality Improvement: Questionnaire Reliability and Validity." *Med Care* 31, no. 9 (Sep 1993): 834-45.

Carpenter, L. M., A. J. Swerdlow, and N. T. Fear. "Mortality of Doctors in Different Specialties: Findings from a Cohort of 20000 Nhs Hospital Consultants." *Occup Environ Med* 54, no. 6 (Jun 1997): 388-95.

Carver, C. S., M. F. Scheier, and J. K. Weintraub. "Assessing Coping Strategies: A Theoretically Based Approach." *J Pers Soc Psychol* 56, no. 2 (Feb 1989): 267-83.

Center, C., M. Davis, T. Detre, D. E. Ford, W. Hansbrough, H. Hendin, J. Laszlo, *et al.* "Confronting Depression and Suicide in Physicians: A Consensus Statement." *JAMA* 289, no. 23 (Jun 18 2003): 3161-6.

Centre, Survey Coordination. "2019 Nhs Staff Survey." National Health Service England. Last modified February 2020. https://www.

nhsstaffsurveyresults.com/wp-content/uploads/2020/01/ P3255_ST19_National-briefing_FINAL_V2.pdf.

Chan, B.; Cochrane, D. *Measuring Patient Harm in Canadian Hospitals. With What Can Be Done to Improve Patient Safety?* Ottawa, ON: Canadian Institute for Health Information, Canadian Patient Safety Institute. 2016.

Chan, Benjamin T. B. "From Perceived Surplus to Perceived Shortage: What Happened to Canadaís Physician Workforce in the 1990s?" (2002). https://secure.cihi.ca/free_products/chanjun02. pdf.

Chiesa, A., and P. Malinowski. "Mindfulness-Based Approaches: Are They All the Same?". *J Clin Psychol* 67, no. 4 (Apr 2011): 404-24.

Chioqueta, Andrea P., and Tore C. Stiles. "Personality Traits and the Development of Depression, Hopelessness, and Suicide Ideation." *Personality and Individual Differences* 38, no. 6 (2005/04/01/ 2005): 1283-91.

Colleges, American Association of Medical. "Figure 18. Percentage of All Active Physicians by Race/Ethnicity, 2018." Accessed January 24, 2021. https://www.aamc.org/data-reports/workforce/interactive-data/figure-18-percentage-all-active-physicians-race/ ethnicity-2018.

Committee, House of Commons Health. "Sixth Report Patient Safety." Accessed November 7, 2021. https://publications.parliament. uk/pa/cm200809/cmselect/cmhealth/151/15106.htm#a2.

Committee, Physician Health Monitoring. "Substance Use and Behavioural Disorders Definitions." College of Physicians & Surgeons of Alberta. Last modified June 2014. http://www.cpsa.ca/physician-health-monitoring-program-phmp/phmp-policies/definitions/#:~:text=Canadian%20Society%20of%20Addiction%20Medicine,psychological%2C%20social%20and%20spiritual%20manifestations.

Cousin, G., M. Schmid Mast, and N. Jaunin-Stalder. "When Physician-Expressed Uncertainty Leads to Patient Dissatisfaction: A Gender Study." *Med Educ* 47, no. 9 (Sep 2013): 923-31.

Dall'Ora, C., P. Griffiths, J. Ball, M. Simon, and L. H. Aiken. "Association of 12 H Shifts and Nurses' Job Satisfaction, Burnout and Intention to Leave: Findings from a Cross-Sectional Study of 12 European Countries." *BMJ Open* 5, no. 9 (Aug 23 2015): e008331.

Dandar, V.M.; Lautenberger, D.M. "Exploring Faculty Salary Equity at U.S. Medical Schools by Gender and Race/Ethnicity." Washington, D.C.: Association of American Medical Colleges, 2021.

Decety, J.; Lamm, C. "Empathy Versus Personal Distress: Recent Evidence from Social Neuroscience." Chap. 15 In *The Social Neuroscience of Empathy*, edited by Jean; Ickes Decety, William 199-213: The MIT Press, 2009.

DeShong, H. L., R. P. Tucker, V. M. O'Keefe, S. N. Mullins-Sweatt, and L. R. Wingate. "Five Factor Model Traits as a Predictor of Suicide Ideation and Interpersonal Suicide Risk in a College Sample." *Psychiatry Res* 226, no. 1 (Mar 30 2015): 217-23.

Dewa, C. S., P. Jacobs, N. X. Thanh, and D. Loong. "An Estimate of the Cost of Burnout on Early Retirement and Reduction in Clinical Hours of Practicing Physicians in Canada." *BMC Health Serv Res* 14 (Jun 13 2014): 254.

Dewa, C. S., D. Loong, S. Bonato, and L. Trojanowski. "The Relationship between Physician Burnout and Quality of Healthcare in Terms of Safety and Acceptability: A Systematic Review." *BMJ Open* 7, no. 6 (Jun 21 2017): e015141.

Donaldson, L. "An Organisation with a Memory." *Clin Med (Lond)* 2, no. 5 (Sep-Oct 2002): 452-7.

Dong, M., F. C. Zhou, S. W. Xu, Q. Zhang, C. H. Ng, G. S. Ungvari, and Y. T. Xiang. "Prevalence of Suicide-Related Behaviors among Physicians: A Systematic Review and Meta-Analysis." *Suicide Life Threat Behav* 50, no. 6 (Dec 2020): 1264-75.

Drapeau, C. W., McIntosh, J. L. (for the American, and Association of Suicidology). "U.S.A. Suicide: 2018 Official Final Data." American Association of Suicidology. Last modified February 12, 2020. http://www.suicidology.org.

Duan, X., X. Ni, L. Shi, L. Zhang, Y. Ye, H. Mu, Z. Li, *et al.* "The Impact of Workplace Violence on Job Satisfaction, Job Burnout, and Turnover Intention: The Mediating Role of Social Support." *Health Qual Life Outcomes* 17, no. 1 (May 30 2019): 93.

Dunn, P. M., B. B. Arnetz, J. F. Christensen, and L. Homer. "Meeting the Imperative to Improve Physician Well-Being: Assessment of an Innovative Program." *J Gen Intern Med* 22, no. 11 (Nov 2007): 1544-52.

Dutheil, F., C. Aubert, B. Pereira, M. Dambrun, F. Moustafa, M. Mermillod, J. S. Baker, *et al.* "Suicide among Physicians and Health-Care Workers: A Systematic Review and Meta-Analysis." *PLoS One* 14, no. 12 (2019): e0226361.

Dweck, C. S. "Mindsets and Human Nature: Promoting Change in the Middle East, the Schoolyard, the Racial Divide, and Willpower." *Am Psychol* 67, no. 8 (Nov 2012): 614-22.

Dyrbye, L. N., T. D. Shanafelt, P. R. Gill, D. V. Satele, and C. P. West. "Effect of a Professional Coaching Intervention on the Well-Being and Distress of Physicians: A Pilot Randomized Clinical Trial." *JAMA Intern Med* 179, no. 10 (Oct 1 2019): 1406-14.

Dyrbye, L. N., M. R. Thomas, F. S. Massie, D. V. Power, A. Eacker, W. Harper, S. Durning, *et al.* "Burnout and Suicidal Ideation among U.S. Medical Students." *Ann Intern Med* 149, no. 5 (Sep 2 2008): 334-41.

Dyrbye, L. N.; Shanafelt, T. D.; Sinsky, C. A.; Cipriano, P. F.; Bhatt J.; Ommaya, A.; West, C. P.; Meyers, D. "Burnout among Health Care Professionals: A Call to Explore and Address This Underrecognized Threat to Safe, High-Quality Care." National Academy of Medicine. Last modified July 5, 2017. https://nam.edu/burnout-among-health-care-professionals-a-call-to-explore-and-address-this-underrecognized-threat-to-safe-high-quality-care/.

Edward, K. L., J. Stephenson, K. Ousey, S. Lui, P. Warelow, and J. A. Giandinoto. "A Systematic Review and Meta-Analysis of Factors That Relate to Aggression Perpetrated against Nurses by Patients/Relatives or Staff." *J Clin Nurs* 25, no. 3-4 (Feb 2016): 289-99.

Elliot, Lisa, Jonathon Tan, and Sarah Norris. *The Mental Health of Doctors: A Systematic Literature Review.* Hawthorn West, Vic.: Beyondblue, 2010.

Employers, NHS. "National Engagement Service." Last modified August 17, 2017. https://www.nhsemployers.org/engagement-and-networks/nhs-employers-engagement-service.

———. "The Relationship between Staff Engagement and Patient Experience." Last modified November 2018. https://www.nhsemployers.org/-/media/Employers/Publications/Staff-engagement/IES-NE-case-studies/Common-themes.pdf.

———. "What We Do." Last modified June 26, 2018. https://www.nhsemployers.org/about-us/what-we-do.

England, Health Education. "Advanced Practice." Accessed April 1, 2021. https://www.hee.nhs.uk/our-work/advanced-clinical-practice.

Enns, M. W., and B. J. Cox. "Personality Dimensions and Depression: Review and Commentary." *Can J Psychiatry* 42, no. 3 (Apr 1997): 274-84.

Epstein, E. G., P. B. Whitehead, C. Prompahakul, L. R. Thacker, and A. B. Hamric. "Enhancing Understanding of Moral Distress: The Measure of Moral Distress for Health Care Professionals." *AJOB Empir Bioeth* 10, no. 2 (Apr-Jun 2019): 113-24.

Escuriex, Brittany F., and Elise E. Labbé. "Health Care Providers' Mindfulness and Treatment Outcomes: A Critical Review of the Research Literature." *Mindfulness* 2, no. 4 (2011/12/01 2011): 242-53.

Flett, Gordon L., and Paul L. Hewitt. "A Proposed Framework for Preventing Perfectionism and Promoting Resilience and Mental Health among Vulnerable Children and Adolescents ". *Psychology in the Schools* 51, no. 9 (11// 2014): 899-912.

Folkman, S., and R. S. Lazarus. "An Analysis of Coping in a Middle-Aged Community Sample." *J Health Soc Behav* 21, no. 3 (Sep 1980): 219-39.

Frank, Erica, Holly Biola, and Carol A. Burnett. "Mortality Rates and Causes among U.S. Physicians." *American Journal of Preventive Medicine* 19, no. 3 (2000): 155-59.

Fridner, A., K. Belkic, M. Marini, D. Minucci, L. Pavan, and K. Schenck-Gustafsson. "Survey on Recent Suicidal Ideation among Female University Hospital Physicians in Sweden and Italy (the Houpe Study): Cross-Sectional Associations with Work Stressors." *Gend Med* 6, no. 1 (Apr 2009): 314-28.

Fridner, A., K. Belkic, D. Minucci, L. Pavan, M. Marini, B. Pingel, G. Putoto, *et al.* "Work Environment and Recent Suicidal Thoughts among Male University Hospital Physicians in Sweden and Italy: The Health and Organization among University Hospital Physicians in Europe (Houpe) Study." *Gend Med* 8, no. 4 (Aug 2011): 269-79.

Garcia, L. C., T. D. Shanafelt, C. P. West, C. A. Sinsky, M. T. Trockel, L. Nedelec, Y. A. Maldonado, *et al.* "Burnout, Depression, Career Satisfaction, and Work-Life Integration by Physician Race/Ethnicity." *JAMA Netw Open* 3, no. 8 (Aug 3 2020): e2012762.

Gittell, J. H., M. Godfrey, and J. Thistlethwaite. "Interprofessional Collaborative Practice and Relational Coordination: Improving Healthcare through Relationships." *J Interprof Care* 27, no. 3 (May 2013): 210-3.

Givens, Jane L., and Jennifer Tjia. "Depressed Medical Students' Use of Mental Health Services and Barriers to Use." *Academic Medicine* 77, no. 9 (2002).

Gleichgerrcht, E., and J. Decety. "Empathy in Clinical Practice: How Individual Dispositions, Gender, and Experience Moderate Empathic Concern, Burnout, and Emotional Distress in Physicians." *PLoS One* 8, no. 4 (2013): e61526.

Goitein, L., T. D. Shanafelt, J. E. Wipf, C. G. Slatore, and A. L. Back. "The Effects of Work-Hour Limitations on Resident Well-Being, Patient Care, and Education in an Internal Medicine Residency Program." *Arch Intern Med* 165, no. 22 (Dec 12-26 2005): 2601-6.

Gold, K. J., L. B. Andrew, E. B. Goldman, and T. L. Schwenk. ""I Would Never Want to Have a Mental Health Diagnosis on My Record": A Survey of Female Physicians on Mental Health Diagnosis, Treatment, and Reporting." *Gen Hosp Psychiatry* 43 (Nov - Dec 2016): 51-57.

Gold, K. J., A. Sen, and T. L. Schwenk. "Details on Suicide among Us Physicians: Data from the National Violent Death Reporting System." *Gen Hosp Psychiatry* 35, no. 1 (Jan-Feb 2013): 45-9.

Gold, Katherine J, Elizabeth R Shih, Edward B Goldman, and Thomas L Schwenk. "Do Us Medical Licensing Applications Treat Mental and Physical Illness Equivalently?". *Fam Med* 49, no. 6 (2017): 464-7.

Gong, Yanhong, Tieguang Han, Xiaoxv Yin, Guoan Yang, Runsen Zhuang, Yuqi Chen, and Zuxun Lu. "Prevalence of Depressive Symptoms and Work-Related Risk Factors among Nurses in

Public Hospitals in Southern China: A Cross-Sectional Study." *Scientific Reports* 4, no. 1 (2014/11/27 2014): 7109.

Goyal, M., S. Singh, E. M. Sibinga, N. F. Gould, A. Rowland-Seymour, R. Sharma, Z. Berger, *et al.* "Meditation Programs for Psychological Stress and Well-Being: A Systematic Review and Meta-Analysis." *JAMA Intern Med* 174, no. 3 (Mar 2014): 357-68.

Grayson, M. S., D. A. Newton, and L. F. Thompson. "Payback Time: The Associations of Debt and Income with Medical Student Career Choice." *Med Educ* 46, no. 10 (Oct 2012): 983-91.

Gregory, S. T., T. Menser, and B. T. Gregory. "An Organizational Intervention to Reduce Physician Burnout." *J Healthc Manag* 63, no. 5 (Sep-Oct 2018): 338-52.

Grocott, H. P., and G. L. Bryson. "The Physician at Risk: Disruptive Behaviour, Burnout, Addiction, and Suicide." *Can J Anaesth* 64, no. 2 (Feb 2017): 119-21.

Groenewold, M. R., R. F. R. Sarmiento, K. Vanoli, W. Raudabaugh, S. Nowlin, and A. Gomaa. "Workplace Violence Injury in 106 Us Hospitals Participating in the Occupational Health Safety Network (Ohsn), 2012-2015." *Am J Ind Med* 61, no. 2 (Feb 2018): 157-66.

Gross, James J. "The Emerging Field of Emotion Regulation: An Integrative Review." *Review of General Psychology* 2, no. 3 (1998): 271-99.

Halbesleben, J. R., and C. Rathert. "Linking Physician Burnout and Patient Outcomes: Exploring the Dyadic Relationship between

Physicians and Patients." *Health Care Manage Rev* 33, no. 1 (Jan-Mar 2008): 29-39.

Halpern, J. *From Detached Concern to Empathy: Humanizing Medical Practice.* Oxford University Press, USA, 2001.

Halpern, J. L. "Beyond "Detached Concern": The Cognitive and Ethical Function of Emotions in Medical Practice." Yale University, 1993.

Halter, M. J., D. G. Rolin, M. Adamaszek, M. C. Ladenheim, and B. F. Hutchens. "State Nursing Licensure Questions About Mental Illness and Compliance with the Americans with Disabilities Act." *J Psychosoc Nurs Ment Health Serv* 57, no. 8 (Aug 1 2019): 17-22.

Hamric, A. B., and L. J. Blackhall. "Nurse-Physician Perspectives on the Care of Dying Patients in Intensive Care Units: Collaboration, Moral Distress, and Ethical Climate." *Crit Care Med* 35, no. 2 (Feb 2007): 422-9.

Han, S., T. D. Shanafelt, C. A. Sinsky, K. M. Awad, L. N. Dyrbye, L. C. Fiscus, M. Trockel, and J. Goh. "Estimating the Attributable Cost of Physician Burnout in the United States." *Ann Intern Med* 170, no. 11 (Jun 4 2019): 784-90.

Hauck, K. D., S. Wang, C. Vincent, and P. C. Smith. "Healthy Life-Years Lost and Excess Bed-Days Due to 6 Patient Safety Incidents: Empirical Evidence from English Hospitals." *Med Care* 55, no. 2 (Feb 2017): 125-30.

Havaei, F., M. MacPhee, and S. E. Lee. "The Effect of Violence Prevention Strategies on Perceptions of Workplace Safety: A Study of

Medical-Surgical and Mental Health Nurses." *J Adv Nurs* 75, no. 8 (Aug 2019): 1657-66.

Havens, D. S., J. H. Gittell, and J. Vasey. "Impact of Relational Coordination on Nurse Job Satisfaction, Work Engagement and Burnout: Achieving the Quadruple Aim." *J Nurs Adm* 48, no. 3 (Mar 2018): 132-40.

Hawton, K., A. Clements, C. Sakarovitch, S. Simkin, and J. J. Deeks. "Suicide in Doctors: A Study of Risk According to Gender, Seniority and Specialty in Medical Practitioners in England and Wales, 1979-1995." *J Epidemiol Community Health* 55, no. 5 (May 2001): 296-300.

Health, National Institute of Mental. "Major Depression." Last modified October 2021. https://www.nimh.nih.gov/health/statistics/major-depression.

Hill, Andrew P., and Thomas Curran. "Multidimensional Perfectionism and Burnout:A Meta-Analysis." *Personality and Social Psychology Review* 20, no. 3 (2016): 269-88.

Holden, R. J., M. C. Scanlon, N. R. Patel, R. Kaushal, K. H. Escoto, R. L. Brown, S. J. Alper, *et al.* "A Human Factors Framework and Study of the Effect of Nursing Workload on Patient Safety and Employee Quality of Working Life." *BMJ Qual Saf* 20, no. 1 (Jan 2011): 15-24.

Implicit, Project. "Project Implicit." Accessed June 16, 2020. https://implicit.harvard.edu/implicit/.

Institute of, Medicine. *To Err Is Human: Building a Safer Health System* [in English]. Edited by T. Kohn Linda, M. Corrigan Janet and

S. Donaldson Molla Washington, DC: The National Academies Press, 2000. doi:10.17226/9728.

Jakobsson, J., M. Axelsson, and K. Ormon. "The Face of Workplace Violence: Experiences of Healthcare Professionals in Surgical Hospital Wards." *Nurs Res Pract* 2020 (2020): 1854387.

Jena, A. B., A. R. Olenski, and D. M. Blumenthal. "Sex Differences in Physician Salary in Us Public Medical Schools." *JAMA Intern Med* 176, no. 9 (Sep 1 2016): 1294-304.

Johnson, K. "Stressed Med Students at High Risk for Later Depression." Medscape. Accessed October 10, 2021. https://www.medscape.com/viewarticle/773650.

Jones, C. B. "The Costs of Nurse Turnover, Part 2: Application of the Nursing Turnover Cost Calculation Methodology." *J Nurs Adm* 35, no. 1 (Jan 2005): 41-9.

———. "Revisiting Nurse Turnover Costs: Adjusting for Inflation." *J Nurs Adm* 38, no. 1 (Jan 2008): 11-8.

Jones, G. M., N. A. Roe, L. Louden, and C. R. Tubbs. "Factors Associated with Burnout among Us Hospital Clinical Pharmacy Practitioners: Results of a Nationwide Pilot Survey." *Hosp Pharm* 52, no. 11 (Dec 2017): 742-51.

Jones, J. T. R., C. S. North, S. Vogel-Scibilia, M. F. Myers, and R. R. Owen. "Medical Licensure Questions About Mental Illness and Compliance with the Americans with Disabilities Act." *J Am Acad Psychiatry Law* 46, no. 4 (Dec 2018): 458-71.

Kalmoe, M. C., M. B. Chapman, J. A. Gold, and A. M. Giedinghagen. "Physician Suicide: A Call to Action." *Mo Med* 116, no. 3 (May-Jun 2019): 211-16.

Kane, L. "Medscape National Physician Burnout & Suicide Report 2020: The Generational Divide." Medscape. Accessed April 4, 2021. https://www.medscape.com/slideshow/2020-lifestyle-burnout-6012460.

Kang, E. K., H. S. Lihm, and E. H. Kong. "Association of Intern and Resident Burnout with Self-Reported Medical Errors." *Korean J Fam Med* 34, no. 1 (Jan 2013): 36-42.

Keeton, K., D. E. Fenner, T. R. Johnson, and R. A. Hayward. "Predictors of Physician Career Satisfaction, Work-Life Balance, and Burnout." *Obstet Gynecol* 109, no. 4 (Apr 2007): 949-55.

Kenna, G. A., and M. D. Wood. "Alcohol Use by Healthcare Professionals." *Drug Alcohol Depend* 75, no. 1 (Jul 15 2004): 107-16.

Khan, N., A. Palepu, P. Dodek, A. Salmon, H. Leitch, S. Ruzycki, A. Townson, and D. Lacaille. "Cross-Sectional Survey on Physician Burnout During the Covid-19 Pandemic in Vancouver, Canada: The Role of Gender, Ethnicity and Sexual Orientation." *BMJ Open* 11, no. 5 (May 10 2021): e050380.

Kim, H., J. S. Kim, K. Choe, Y. Kwak, and J. S. Song. "Mediating Effects of Workplace Violence on the Relationships between Emotional Labour and Burnout among Clinical Nurses." *J Adv Nurs* 74, no. 10 (Oct 2018): 2331-39.

Ko, D. T., A. Chu, P. C. Austin, S. Johnston, B. K. Nallamothu, I. Roifman, N. Tusevljak, J. A. Udell, and E. Frank. "Comparison of Cardiovascular Risk Factors and Outcomes among Practicing Physicians Vs the General Population in Ontario, Canada." *JAMA Netw Open* 2, no. 11 (Nov 1 2019): e1915983.

Kobayashi, Y., M. Oe, T. Ishida, M. Matsuoka, H. Chiba, and N. Uchimura. "Workplace Violence and Its Effects on Burnout and Secondary Traumatic Stress among Mental Healthcare Nurses in Japan." *Int J Environ Res Public Health* 17, no. 8 (Apr 16 2020).

Koutsimani, P., A. Montgomery, and K. Georganta. "The Relationship between Burnout, Depression, and Anxiety: A Systematic Review and Meta-Analysis." *Front Psychol* 10 (2019): 284.

Kriakous, S. A., K. A. Elliott, C. Lamers, and R. Owen. "The Effectiveness of Mindfulness-Based Stress Reduction on the Psychological Functioning of Healthcare Professionals: A Systematic Review." *Mindfulness (N Y)* (Sep 24 2020): 1-28.

Kuhn, C. M., and E. M. Flanagan. "Self-Care as a Professional Imperative: Physician Burnout, Depression, and Suicide." *Can J Anaesth* 64, no. 2 (Feb 2017): 158-68.

Kumpfer, K.L. "Factors and Processes Contributing to Resilience: The Resilience Framework." In *Resilience and Development: Positive Life Adaptations*, edited by M.D.; Johnson Glantz, J.L., 179-224. New York: Kluwer Academic Publishers, 1999.

Laeeque, Syed Harris, Atif Bilal, Samreen Babar, Zoya Khan, and Saif Ul Rahman. "How Patient-Perpetrated Workplace Violence Leads to Turnover Intention among Nurses: The Mediating Mechanism of Occupational Stress and Burnout." *Journal of Aggression, Maltreatment & Trauma* 27, no. 1 (2018/01/02 2018): 96-118.

Lampert, Bettina, and Jürgen Glaser. "Detached Concern in Client Interaction and Burnout." *International Journal of Stress Management* 25, no. 2 (2018): 129-43.

Lastovkova, A., M. Carder, H. M. Rasmussen, L. Sjoberg, G. J. Groene, R. Sauni, J. Vevoda, *et al.* "Burnout Syndrome as an Occupational Disease in the European Union: An Exploratory Study." *Ind Health* 56, no. 2 (Apr 7 2018): 160-65.

Leape, Lucian L. "Medical Errors and Patient Safety." Chap. 5 In *The Trust Crisis in Healthcare: Causes, Consequences, and Cures*, edited by David A. Shore, 60-61. New York: Oxford University Press, 2007.

Leary, M.R., and R.H. Hoyle. *Handbook of Individual Differences in Social Behavior*. Guilford Publications, 2009.

Lee, B.Y. "Time to Stop Labeling Physicians as Providers." Forbes. Accessed March 31, 2021. https://www.forbes.com/sites/brucelee/2019/05/05/time-to-stop-labeling-physicians-as-providers/.

Lee, P. T., J. Loh, G. Sng, J. Tung, and K. K. Yeo. "Empathy and Burnout: A Study on Residents from a Singapore Institution." *Singapore Med J* 59, no. 1 (Jan 2018): 50-54.

Lefebvre, L. G., and I. M. Kaufmann. "The Identification and Management of Substance Use Disorders in Anesthesiologists." *Can J Anaesth* 64, no. 2 (Feb 2017): 211-18.

Leiter, Michael P., Phyllis Harvie, and Cindy Frizzell. "The Correspondence of Patient Satisfaction and Nurse Burnout." *Social Science & Medicine* 47, no. 10 (1998/11/01/ 1998): 1611-17.

Letvak, S., C. J. Ruhm, and T. McCoy. "Depression in Hospital-Employed Nurses." *Clin Nurse Spec* 26, no. 3 (May-Jun 2012): 177-82.

Li, B., L. Bruyneel, W. Sermeus, K. Van den Heede, K. Matawie, L. Aiken, and E. Lesaffre. "Group-Level Impact of Work Environment Dimensions on Burnout Experiences among Nurses: A Multivariate Multilevel Probit Model." *Int J Nurs Stud* 50, no. 2 (Feb 2013): 281-91.

Li, M., J. Liu, J. Zheng, K. Liu, J. Wang, A. Miner Ross, X. Liu, *et al.* "The Relationship of Workplace Violence and Nurse Outcomes: Gender Difference Study on a Propensity Score Matched Sample." *J Adv Nurs* 76, no. 2 (Feb 2020): 600-10.

Lindeman, S., E. Laara, H. Hakko, and J. Lonnqvist. "A Systematic Review on Gender-Specific Suicide Mortality in Medical Doctors." *Br J Psychiatry* 168, no. 3 (Mar 1996): 274-9.

Linzer, M., and E. Harwood. "Gendered Expectations: Do They Contribute to High Burnout among Female Physicians?". *J Gen Intern Med* 33, no. 6 (Jun 2018): 963-65.

Locke, T. "Medscape Uk Doctors' Burnout & Lifestyle Survey 2020." Medscape. Accessed April 4, 2021. https://www.medscape.com/slideshow/uk-doctors-burnout-2020-6013312.

Lyubomirsky, Sonja, Kennon M. Sheldon, and David Schkade. "Pursuing Happiness: The Architecture of Sustainable Change." *Review of General Psychology* 9, no. 2 (2005): 111-31.

Mahan, C. E., M. T. Holdsworth, S. M. Welch, M. Borrego, and A. C. Spyropoulos. "Deep-Vein Thrombosis: A United States Cost Model for a Preventable and Costly Adverse Event." *Thromb Haemost* 106, no. 3 (Sep 2011): 405-15.

Makary, Martin A., and Michael Daniel. "Medical Error—the Third Leading Cause of Death in the Us." *BMJ* 353 (2016): i2139.

Martins Pereira, S., C. M. Teixeira, A. S. Carvalho, P. Hernandez-Marrero, and InPalIn. "Compared to Palliative Care, Working in Intensive Care More Than Doubles the Chances of Burnout: Results from a Nationwide Comparative Study." *PLoS One* 11, no. 9 (2016): e0162340.

Maruff, Paul, Marina G. Falleti, Alex Collie, David Darby, and Michael McStephen. "Fatigue-Related Impairment in the Speed, Accuracy and Variability of Psychomotor Performance: Comparison with Blood Alcohol Levels." *Journal of Sleep Research* 14, no. 1 (2005): 21-27.

Maslach, C., Jackson, S.E., and Leiter, M.P. *Maslach Burnout Inventory*. 3 ed. Palo Alto, California: Consulting Psychologists Press, 1996.

Maslach, C., and M. P. Leiter. "Understanding the Burnout Experience: Recent Research and Its Implications for Psychiatry." *World Psychiatry* 15, no. 2 (Jun 2016): 103-11.

Maslach, C., W. B. Schaufeli, and M. P. Leiter. "Job Burnout." *Annu Rev Psychol* 52 (2001): 397-422.

Maslach, Christina. "The Client Role in Staff Burn-Out." *Journal of Social Issues* 34, no. 4 (1978): 111-24.

———. "Finding Solutions to the Problem of Burnout." *Consulting Psychology Journal: Practice and Research* 69, no. 2 (2017): 143-52.

Maslow, A. H. "A Theory of Human Motivation." *Psychological Review* 50, no. 4 (1943): 370-96.

Mata, D. A., M. A. Ramos, N. Bansal, R. Khan, C. Guille, E. Di Angelantonio, and S. Sen. "Prevalence of Depression and Depressive Symptoms among Resident Physicians: A Systematic Review and Meta-Analysis." *JAMA* 314, no. 22 (Dec 8 2015): 2373-83.

McAbee, J. H., B. T. Ragel, S. McCartney, G. M. Jones, L. M. Michael, 2nd, M. DeCuypere, J. S. Cheng, F. A. Boop, and P. Klimo, Jr. "Factors Associated with Career Satisfaction and Burnout among Us Neurosurgeons: Results of a Nationwide Survey." *J Neurosurg* 123, no. 1 (Jul 2015): 161-73.

McHugh, M. D., and C. Ma. "Wage, Work Environment, and Staffing: Effects on Nurse Outcomes." *Policy Polit Nurs Pract* 15, no. 3-4 (Aug-Nov 2014): 72-80.

McLellan, A. T., G. S. Skipper, M. Campbell, and R. L. DuPont. "Five Year Outcomes in a Cohort Study of Physicians Treated for Substance Use Disorders in the United States." *BMJ* 337 (Nov 4 2008): a2038.

McMurray, J. E., M. Linzer, T. R. Konrad, J. Douglas, R. Shugerman, and K. Nelson. "The Work Lives of Women Physicians Results from the Physician Work Life Study. The Sgim Career Satisfaction Study Group." [In eng]. *Journal of general internal medicine* 15, no. 6 (2000): 372-80.

Medicine, National Library of. "Greek Medicine." Last modified February 7, 2012. https://www.nlm.nih.gov/hmd/greek/greek_oath.html.

Melnick, E. R., L. N. Dyrbye, C. A. Sinsky, M. Trockel, C. P. West, L. Ned-elec, M. A. Tutty, and T. Shanafelt. "The Association between Perceived Electronic Health Record Usability and Professional Burnout among Us Physicians." *Mayo Clin Proc* 95, no. 3 (Mar 2020): 476-87.

Menon, N. K., T. D. Shanafelt, C. A. Sinsky, M. Linzer, L. Carlasare, K. J. S. Brady, M. J. Stillman, and M. T. Trockel. "Association of Physician Burnout with Suicidal Ideation and Medical Errors." *JAMA Netw Open* 3, no. 12 (Dec 1 2020): e2028780.

Merriam-Webster. "Compassion." Merriam-Webster.com Dictionary. Accessed November 15, 2020. https://www.merriam-webster.com/dictionary/compassion.

———. "Empathy." Merriam-Webster.com Dictionary. Accessed November 15, 2020. https://www.merriam-webster.com/dictionary/empathy.

———. "Overachiever." Merriam-Webster.com Dictionary. Accessed May 3, 2021. https://www.merriam-webster.com/dictionary/overachiever.

———. "Proof." Merriam-Webster.com Dictionary. Accessed May 3, 2021. https://www.merriam-webster.com/dictionary/proof.

———. "Resilience." Merriam-Webster.com Dictionary. Accessed November 11, 2020. https://www.merriam-webster.com/dictionary/resilience.

———. "Stereotype." Merriam-Webster.com Dictionary. Accessed April 18, 2021. https://www.merriam-webster.com/dictionary/stereotype.

Myers, D. G. "The Self in a Social World." Chap. 2 In *Social Psychology*, 56-58. New York: McGraw-Hill, 2012.

Myers, M., and C. Fine. "Suicide in Physicians: Toward Prevention." *MedGenMed* 5, no. 4 (Oct 21 2003): 11.

National Academies of Sciences, Engineering, and Medicine; National Academy of Medicine; Committee on Systems Approaches to Improve Patient Care by Supporting Clinician Well-Being. "Taking Action against Clinician Burnout: A Systems Approach to Professional Well-Being." In *Taking Action against Clinician Burnout: A Systems Approach to Professional Well-Being*. Washington (DC): National Academies Press, 2019.

Nedrow, A., N. A. Steckler, and J. Hardman. "Physician Resilience and Burnout: Can You Make the Switch?". *Fam Pract Manag* 20, no. 1 (Jan-Feb 2013): 25-30.

Network, ADA National. "What Is the Americans with Disabilities Act (Ada)?" Accessed May 26, 2021. https://adata.org/learn-about-ada.

Noland, S. T., H. Taipale, J. I. Mahmood, and R. Tyssen. "Analysis of Career Stage, Gender, and Personality and Workplace Violence in a 20-Year Nationwide Cohort of Physicians in Norway." *JAMA Netw Open* 4, no. 6 (Jun 1 2021): e2114749.

Ohler, M. C., M. S. Kerr, and D. A. Forbes. "Depression in Nurses." *Can J Nurs Res* 42, no. 3 (Sep 2010): 66-82.

Oreskovich, M. R., T. Shanafelt, L. N. Dyrbye, L. Tan, W. Sotile, D. Satele, C. P. West, J. Sloan, and S. Boone. "The Prevalence of Substance

Use Disorders in American Physicians." *Am J Addict* 24, no. 1 (Jan 2015): 30-8.

Organization, World Health. "10 Facts on Patient Safety." Last modified August 2019. https://www.who.int/news-room/photo-story/photo-story-detail/10-facts-on-patient-safety.

———. "The Conceptual Framework for the International Classification for Patient Safety." Accessed July 4, 2021. https://www.who.int/publications/i/item/the-conceptual-framework-for-the-international-classification-for-patient-safety-(icps).

———. "Depression." Last modified September 13, 2021. https://www.who.int/news-room/fact-sheets/detail/depression.

———. "Icd-10 Version:2019." Accessed March 25, 2020. https://icd.who.int/browse10/2019/en#/Z73.

———. "Icd-11 for Mortality and Morbidity Statistics." Accessed March 25, 2020. https://icd.who.int/browse11/l-m/en#/http://id.who.int/icd/entity/129180281.

———. "International Classification of Diseases (Icd) Revision." Accessed May 1, 2020. https://www.who.int/classifications/icd/revision/icd11faq/en/.

———. "Reporting and Learning Systems." Accessed May 22, 2020. https://www.who.int/patientsafety/topics/reporting-learning/en/.

Panagioti, M., E. Panagopoulou, P. Bower, G. Lewith, E. Kontopantelis, C. Chew-Graham, S. Dawson, *et al.* "Controlled Interventions to Reduce Burnout in Physicians: A Systematic Review and Meta-Analysis." *JAMA Intern Med* 177, no. 2 (Feb 1 2017): 195-205.

Perrin, M., C. L. Vandeleur, E. Castelao, S. Rothen, J. Glaus, P. Vollen-
weider, and M. Preisig. "Determinants of the Development of
Post-Traumatic Stress Disorder, in the General Population." *Soc
Psychiatry Psychiatr Epidemiol* 49, no. 3 (Mar 2014): 447-57.

Peterson, C., D. M. Stone, S. M. Marsh, P. K. Schumacher, H. M. Ties-
man, W. L. McIntosh, C. N. Lokey, *et al.* "Suicide Rates by Major
Occupational Group - 17 States, 2012 and 2015." *MMWR Morb
Mortal Wkly Rep* 67, no. 45 (Nov 16 2018): 1253-60.

Petitta, Laura, Lixin Jiang, and Charmine E.J. Härtel. "Emotional Contagion and Burnout among Nurses and Doctors: Do Joy and Anger from Different Sources of Stakeholders Matter?". *Stress and
Health* 33, no. 4 (2017): 358-69.

Philibert, I., P. Friedmann, W. T. Williams, and Acgme Work Group on
Resident Duty Hours. Accreditation Council for Graduate Med-
ical Education. "New Requirements for Resident Duty Hours."
JAMA 288, no. 9 (Sep 4 2002): 1112-4.

Phillips, J. "The Impact of Debt on Young Family Physicians: Unan-
swered Questions with Critical Implications." *J Am Board Fam
Med* 29, no. 2 (Mar-Apr 2016): 177-9.

Phillips, J. P. "Workplace Violence against Health Care Workers in the
United States." *N Engl J Med* 374, no. 17 (Apr 28 2016): 1661-9.

Physicians, American Society of. "Support for Assistant Physician Licenses." Accessed June 8, 2021 https://www.linkedin.com/
posts/asphysicians_ap-license-support-statement-activi-
ty-6703677529443631104-DCl-.

Pratt, M., M. Kerr, and C. Wong. "The Impact of Eri, Burnout, and Caring for Sars Patients on Hospital Nurses' Self-Reported Compliance with Infection Control." *Can J Infect Control* 24, no. 3 (Fall 2009): 167-72, 74.

Program, National Resident Matching. "Advance Data Tables 2021 Main Residency Match." Accessed June 3, 2021. https://mk0nrmp3oyqui6wqfm.kinstacdn.com/wp-content/uploads/2021/03/Advance-Data-Tables-2021_Final.pdf.

———. "Charting Outcomes in the Match: International Medical Graduates." Accessed June 14, 2021. https://mk0nrmp3oyqui6wqfm.kinstacdn.com/wp-content/uploads/2020/07/Charting-Outcomes-in-the-Match-2020_IMG_final.pdf.

Psychology, APA Dictionary of. "Hindsight Bias." American Psychology Association. Accessed May 17, 2021. https://dictionary.apa.org/hindsight-bias.

Pulse. "Number of Registered Patients Per Gp Rises to Almost 2,100." Last modified July 11, 2019. https://www.pulsetoday.co.uk/news/workload/number-of-registered-patients-per-gp-rises-to-almost-2100/.

Quillian, L. , A. Heath, D. Pager, A.H. Midtbøen, F. Fleischmann, and O. Hexel. "Do Some Countries Discriminate More Than Others? Evidence from 97 Field Experiments of Racial Discrimination in Hiring." *Sociological Science* 6, no. 18 (2019): 467-96.

Rasmussen, V., A. Turnell, P. Butow, I. Juraskova, L. Kirsten, L. Wiener, A. Patenaude, *et al.* "Burnout among Psychosocial Oncologists: An Application and Extension of the Effort-Reward Imbalance Model." *Psychooncology* 25, no. 2 (Feb 2016): 194-202.

Read, E., and H. K. Laschinger. "Correlates of New Graduate Nurses' Experiences of Workplace Mistreatment." *J Nurs Adm* 43, no. 4 (Apr 2013): 221-8.

Reason, J. *Managing the Risks of Organizational Accidents.* Routledge, 2016.

Rees, C., L. Wirihana, R. Eley, R. Ossieran-Moisson, and D. Hegney. "The Effects of Occupational Violence on the Well-Being and Resilience of Nurses." *J Nurs Adm* 48, no. 9 (Sep 2018): 452-58.

Reid, R. J., K. Coleman, E. A. Johnson, P. A. Fishman, C. Hsu, M. P. Soman, C. E. Trescott, M. Erikson, and E. B. Larson. "The Group Health Medical Home at Year Two: Cost Savings, Higher Patient Satisfaction, and Less Burnout for Providers." *Health Aff (Millwood)* 29, no. 5 (May 2010): 835-43.

RiskAnalytica. "The Case for Investing in Patient Safety in Canada." (2017). https://www.patientsafetyinstitute.ca/en/toolsResources/Documents/Patient%20Harm%20Awareness%20-%20Ipsos/Risk%20Analytica%202017%20The%20Case%20for%20Investing%20in%20Patient%20Safety%20in%20Canada.pdf.

Robins, Richard W., and Jennifer L. Pals. "Implicit Self-Theories in the Academic Domain: Implications for Goal Orientation, Attributions, Affect, and Self-Esteem Change." *Self and Identity* 1, no. 4 (2002/10/01 2002): 313-36.

Ross, M. "Suicide among Physicians." *Psychiatry Med* 2, no. 3 (Jul 1971): 189-98.

Rotenstein, L. S., M. A. Ramos, M. Torre, J. B. Segal, M. J. Peluso, C. Guille, S. Sen, and D. A. Mata. "Prevalence of Depression, Depressive Symptoms, and Suicidal Ideation among Medical Students: A Systematic Review and Meta-Analysis." *JAMA* 316, no. 21 (Dec 6 2016): 2214-36.

Rushton, C. H., J. Batcheller, K. Schroeder, and P. Donohue. "Burnout and Resilience among Nurses Practicing in High-Intensity Settings." *Am J Crit Care* 24, no. 5 (Sep 2015): 412-20.

Salyers, M. P., K. A. Bonfils, L. Luther, R. L. Firmin, D. A. White, E. L. Adams, and A. L. Rollins. "The Relationship between Professional Burnout and Quality and Safety in Healthcare: A Meta-Analysis." *J Gen Intern Med* 32, no. 4 (Apr 2017): 475-82.

Sargent, Douglas A., Viggo W. Jensen, Thomas A. Petty, and Herbert Raskin. "Preventing Physician Suicide: The Role of Family, Colleagues, and Organized Medicine." *JAMA* 237, no. 2 (1977): 143-45.

Schaufeli, W.B., M.P. Leiter, and C. Maslach. "Burnout: 35 Years of Research and Practice." *Career Development International* 14, no. 3 (2009): 204-20.

Schaufeli, W.B., C. Maslach, and T. Marek. *Professional Burnout: Recent Developments in Theory and Research*. Taylor & Francis, 2017.

Schmid Mast, M., J. A. Hall, and D. L. Roter. "Disentangling Physician Sex and Physician Communication Style: Their Effects on Patient Satisfaction in a Virtual Medical Visit." *Patient Educ Couns* 68, no. 1 (Sep 2007): 16-22.

Schroeder, R., C. M. Brazeau, F. Zackin, S. Rovi, J. Dickey, M. S. Johnson, and S. E. Keller. "Do State Medical Board Applications Violate the Americans with Disabilities Act?". *Acad Med* 84, no. 6 (Jun 2009): 776-81.

Sen, S., H. R. Kranzler, J. H. Krystal, H. Speller, G. Chan, J. Gelernter, and C. Guille. "A Prospective Cohort Study Investigating Factors Associated with Depression During Medical Internship." *Arch Gen Psychiatry* 67, no. 6 (Jun 2010): 557-65.

Service, Canadian Resident Matching. "2021 Carms Forum." Last modified May 31, 2021. https://carms.ca/pdfs/2021-carms-forum.pdf.

———. "Table 1: Summary of Match Results." Accessed November 23, 2021. https://www.carms.ca/wp-content/uploads/2020/05/2020_r1_tbl1e.pdf.

———. "Table 1: Summary of Match Results." Accessed November 23, 2021. https://www.carms.ca/wp-content/uploads/2021/06/r1_tbl1e.pdf.

———. "Table 3: Summary of Positions by School of Residency." Accessed November 23, 2021. https://www.carms.ca/wp-content/uploads/2020/05/2020_r1_tbl3e.pdf.

Shanafelt, T. D., C. M. Balch, G. J. Bechamps, T. Russell, L. Dyrbye, D. Satele, P. Collicott, *et al.* "Burnout and Career Satisfaction among American Surgeons." *Ann Surg* 250, no. 3 (Sep 2009): 463-71.

Shanafelt, T. D., C. M. Balch, L. Dyrbye, G. Bechamps, T. Russell, D. Satele, T. Rummans, *et al.* "Special Report: Suicidal Ideation among American Surgeons." *Arch Surg* 146, no. 1 (Jan 2011): 54-62.

Shanafelt, T. D., L. N. Dyrbye, C. Sinsky, O. Hasan, D. Satele, J. Sloan, and C. P. West. "Relationship between Clerical Burden and Characteristics of the Electronic Environment with Physician Burnout and Professional Satisfaction." *Mayo Clin Proc* 91, no. 7 (Jul 2016): 836-48.

Shanafelt, T. D., L. N. Dyrbye, C. P. West, C. Sinsky, M. Tutty, L. E. Carlasare, H. Wang, and M. Trockel. "Suicidal Ideation and Attitudes Regarding Help Seeking in Us Physicians Relative to the Us Working Population." *Mayo Clin Proc* 96, no. 8 (Aug 2021): 2067-80.

Shanafelt, T. D., W. J. Gradishar, M. Kosty, D. Satele, H. Chew, L. Horn, B. Clark, *et al.* "Burnout and Career Satisfaction among Us Oncologists." *J Clin Oncol* 32, no. 7 (Mar 1 2014): 678-86.

Shanafelt, T. D., C. P. West, C. Sinsky, M. Trockel, M. Tutty, D. V. Satele, L. E. Carlasare, and L. N. Dyrbye. "Changes in Burnout and Satisfaction with Work-Life Integration in Physicians and the General Us Working Population between 2011 and 2017." *Mayo Clin Proc* 94, no. 9 (Sep 2019): 1681-94.

Shanafelt, T. D., C. P. West, J. A. Sloan, P. J. Novotny, G. A. Poland, R. Menaker, T. A. Rummans, and L. N. Dyrbye. "Career Fit and Burnout among Academic Faculty." *Arch Intern Med* 169, no. 10 (May 25 2009): 990-5.

Shanafelt, T., J. Ripp, and M. Trockel. "Understanding and Addressing Sources of Anxiety among Health Care Professionals During the Covid-19 Pandemic." *JAMA* 323, no. 21 (Jun 2 2020): 2133-34.

Shangraw, A. M., J. Silvers, T. Warholak, and N. Vadiei. "Prevalence of Anxiety and Depressive Symptoms among Pharmacy Students." *Am J Pharm Educ* 85, no. 2 (Feb 2021): 8166.

Shapiro, D. E., C. Duquette, L. M. Abbott, T. Babineau, A. Pearl, and P. Haidet. "Beyond Burnout: A Physician Wellness Hierarchy Designed to Prioritize Interventions at the Systems Level." *Am J Med* 132, no. 5 (May 2019): 556-63.

Shea, J. A., D. F. Dinges, D. S. Small, M. Basner, J. Zhu, L. Norton, A. J. Ecker, *et al.* "A Randomized Trial of a Three-Hour Protected Nap Period in a Medicine Training Program: Sleep, Alertness, and Patient Outcomes." *Acad Med* 89, no. 3 (Mar 2014): 452-9.

Shi, J., S. Wang, P. Zhou, L. Shi, Y. Zhang, F. Bai, D. Xue, and X. Zhang. "The Frequency of Patient-Initiated Violence and Its Psychological Impact on Physicians in China: A Cross-Sectional Study." *PLoS One* 10, no. 6 (2015): e0128394.

Shi, L., L. Wang, X. Jia, Z. Li, H. Mu, X. Liu, B. Peng, A. Li, and L. Fan. "Prevalence and Correlates of Symptoms of Post-Traumatic Stress Disorder among Chinese Healthcare Workers Exposed to Physical Violence: A Cross-Sectional Study." *BMJ Open* 7, no. 7 (Aug 1 2017): e016810.

Shin, Hyojung, Yang Park, Jin Ying, Boyoung Kim, Hyunkyung Noh, and Sang Lee. "Relationships between Coping Strategies and Burnout Symptoms: A Meta-Analytic Approach." *Professional Psychology: Research and Practice* 45 (02/01 2014): 44.

Shojania, Kaveh G., and Mary Dixon-Woods. "Estimating Deaths Due to Medical Error: The Ongoing Controversy and Why It Matters." *BMJ Quality & Safety* 26, no. 5 (2017): 423.

Sinsky, C. A., L. N. Dyrbye, C. P. West, D. Satele, M. Tutty, and T. D. Shanafelt. "Professional Satisfaction and the Career Plans of Us Physicians." [In eng]. *Mayo Clin Proc* 92, no. 11 (Nov 2017): 1625-35.

Skipper, Gregory E., Michael D. Campbell, and Robert L. DuPont. "Anesthesiologists with Substance Use Disorders: A 5-Year Outcome Study from 16 State Physician Health Programs." *Anesthesia & Analgesia* 109, no. 3 (2009): 891-96.

Slawomirski, Luke, Ane Auraaen, and Niek S. Klazinga. "The Economics of Patient Safety: Strengthening a Value-Based Approach to Reducing Patient Harm at National Level." Paper presented at the 2nd Global Ministerial Summit on Patient Safety, Bonn, Germany, 2017.

Snowden, D. J., and M. E. Boone. "A Leader's Framework for Decision Making. A Leader's Framework for Decision Making." *Harv Bus Rev* 85, no. 11 (Nov 2007): 68-76, 149.

Solomon, A. W., C. J. Kirwan, N. D. Alexander, K. Nimako, A. Jurukov, R. J. Forth, T. M. Rahman, and Investigators Prospective Analysis of Renal Compensation for Hypohydration in Exhausted Doctors. "Urine Output on an Intensive Care Unit: Case-Control Study." *BMJ* 341 (Dec 14 2010): c6761.

Stehman, C. R., Z. Testo, R. S. Gershaw, and A. R. Kellogg. "Burnout, Drop out, Suicide: Physician Loss in Emergency Medicine, Part I." *West J Emerg Med* 20, no. 3 (May 2019): 485-94.

Stelnicki, A. M., L. Jamshidi, A. Angehrn, and R. Nicholas Carleton. "Suicidal Behaviors among Nurses in Canada." *Can J Nurs Res* 52, no. 3 (Sep 2020): 226-36.

Suicidology, American Association of. "Warning Signs." Accessed June 3, 2021. http://suicidology.org/resources/warning-signs/.

Sutherland, V. J., and C. L. Cooper. "Identifying Distress among General Practitioners: Predictors of Psychological Ill-Health and Job Dissatisfaction." *Social Science & Medicine* 37, no. 5 (1993/09/01/ 1993): 575-81.

Tak, H. J., F. A. Curlin, and J. D. Yoon. "Association of Intrinsic Motivating Factors and Markers of Physician Well-Being: A National Physician Survey." *J Gen Intern Med* 32, no. 7 (Jul 2017): 739-46.

Tan, Yi Quan, Ziting Wang, Qai Ven Yap, Yiong Huak Chan, Roger C. Ho, Agus Rizal Ardy Hariandy Hamid, Aitor Landaluce-Olavarria, *et al.* "Psychological Health of Surgeons in a Time of Covid-19: A Global Survey." *Annals of Surgery* (2021).

Tawfik, D. S., J. Profit, T. I. Morgenthaler, D. V. Satele, C. A. Sinsky, L. N. Dyrbye, M. A. Tutty, C. P. West, and T. D. Shanafelt. "Physician Burnout, Well-Being, and Work Unit Safety Grades in Relationship to Reported Medical Errors." *Mayo Clin Proc* 93, no. 11 (Nov 2018): 1571-80.

Thomas, L. R., J. A. Ripp, and C. P. West. "Charter on Physician Well-Being." *JAMA* 319, no. 15 (Apr 17 2018): 1541-42.

Treiber, L. A., and J. H. Jones. "Making an Infusion Error: The Second Victims of Infusion Therapy-Related Medication Errors." *J Infus Nurs* 41, no. 3 (May/Jun 2018): 156-63.

Tung, Y. J., K. K. H. Lo, R. C. M. Ho, and W. S. W. Tam. "Prevalence of Depression among Nursing Students: A Systematic Review and Meta-Analysis." *Nurse Educ Today* 63 (Apr 2018): 119-29.

Tyssen, R. "Work and Mental Health in Doctors: A Short Review of Norwegian Studies." *Porto Biomed J* 4, no. 5 (Sep-Oct 2019): e50.

Tyssen, Reidar. "Personality Traits." In *Physician Mental Health and Well-Being: Research and Practice*, edited by Kirk J. Brower and Michelle B. Riba, 211-34. Cham: Springer International Publishing, 2017.

Van Aerde, J.; Gautam, M. . "Leadership Agility in Chaotic Systems." In *Canadian Society of Physician Leaders Covid-19 Bulletin #2*, edited by Canadian Society of Physician Leaders: Canadian Society of Physician Leaders, 2020.

van der Heijden, F., G. Dillingh, A. Bakker, and J. Prins. "Suicidal Thoughts among Medical Residents with Burnout." *Arch Suicide Res* 12, no. 4 (2008): 344-6.

van der Wal, R. A., M. J. Bucx, J. C. Hendriks, G. J. Scheffer, and J. B. Prins. "Psychological Distress, Burnout and Personality Traits in Dutch Anaesthesiologists: A Survey." *Eur J Anaesthesiol* 33, no. 3 (Mar 2016): 179-86.

Van Dongen, H. P., G. Maislin, J. M. Mullington, and D. F. Dinges. "The Cumulative Cost of Additional Wakefulness: Dose-Response Effects on Neurobehavioral Functions and Sleep Physiology from Chronic Sleep Restriction and Total Sleep Deprivation." *Sleep* 26, no. 2 (Mar 15 2003): 117-26.

Velting, Drew M. "Suicidal Ideation and the Five-Factor Model of Personality." *Personality and Individual Differences* 27, no. 5 (1999/11/01/ 1999): 943-52.

von Harscher, H., N. Desmarais, R. Dollinger, S. Grossman, and S. Aldana. "The Impact of Empathy on Burnout in Medical Students: New Findings." *Psychol Health Med* 23, no. 3 (Mar 2018): 295-303.

Walji, M. "Diversity in Medical Education: Data Drought and Socioeconomic Barriers." *CMAJ* 187, no. 1 (Jan 6 2015): 11.

Walker, Matthew. *Why We Sleep*. Harlow, England: Penguin Books, 2018.

Welsh, D. "Predictors of Depressive Symptoms in Female Medical-Surgical Hospital Nurses." *Issues Ment Health Nurs* 30, no. 5 (May 2009): 320-6.

West, C. P., L. N. Dyrbye, C. Sinsky, M. Trockel, M. Tutty, L. Nedelec, L. E. Carlasare, and T. D. Shanafelt. "Resilience and Burnout among Physicians and the General Us Working Population." *JAMA Netw Open* 3, no. 7 (Jul 1 2020): e209385.

West, C. P., T. D. Shanafelt, and J. C. Kolars. "Quality of Life, Burnout, Educational Debt, and Medical Knowledge among Internal Medicine Residents." *JAMA* 306, no. 9 (Sep 7 2011): 952-60.

West, Colin P., Liselotte N. Dyrbye, Patricia J. Erwin, and Tait D. Shanafelt. "Interventions to Prevent and Reduce Physician Burnout: A Systematic Review and Meta-Analysis." *The Lancet* 388, no. 10057 (2016/11/05/ 2016): 2272-81.

White, B., and D. Twiddy. "The State of Family Medicine: 2017." *Fam Pract Manag* 24, no. 1 (Jan/Feb 2017): 26-33.

White, E. M., L. H. Aiken, and M. D. McHugh. "Registered Nurse Burnout, Job Dissatisfaction, and Missed Care in Nursing Homes." *J Am Geriatr Soc* 67, no. 10 (Oct 2019): 2065-71.

Wilkinson, H., R. Whittington, L. Perry, and C. Eames. "Examining the Relationship between Burnout and Empathy in Healthcare Professionals: A Systematic Review." *Burn Res* 6 (Sep 2017): 18-29.

Williamson, A. M., and A. M. Feyer. "Moderate Sleep Deprivation Produces Impairments in Cognitive and Motor Performance Equivalent to Legally Prescribed Levels of Alcohol Intoxication." *Occup Environ Med* 57, no. 10 (Oct 2000): 649-55.

Wilson, R. M., W. B. Runciman, R. W. Gibberd, B. T. Harrison, L. Newby, and J. D. Hamilton. "The Quality in Australian Health Care Study." *Med J Aust* 163, no. 9 (Nov 6 1995): 458-71.

Windover, A. K., K. Martinez, M. B. Mercer, K. Neuendorf, A. Boissy, and M. B. Rothberg. "Correlates and Outcomes of Physician Burnout within a Large Academic Medical Center." *JAMA Intern Med* 178, no. 6 (Jun 1 2018): 856-58.

Wisenberg Brin, Dinah. "Taking the Sting out of Medical School Debt." Association of American Medical Colleges. Last modified April 4, 2017. https://www.aamc.org/news-insights/taking-sting-out-medical-school-debt.

Wolf, Zane Robinson, Joanne F. Serembus, Judy Smetzer, Hedy Cohen, and Michael Cohen. "Responses and Concerns of Healthcare Providers to Medication Errors." *Clinical Nurse Specialist* 14, no. 6 (2000).

WorkSafeBC. "Health Care and Social Services High Risk Strategy." Accessed April 12, 2021. https://www.worksafebc.com/en/about-us/what-we-do/high-risk-strategies/health-care.

Wu, A. W. "Medical Error: The Second Victim. The Doctor Who Makes the Mistake Needs Help Too." *BMJ* 320, no. 7237 (Mar 18 2000): 726-7.

Yaghmour, N. A., T. P. Brigham, T. Richter, R. S. Miller, I. Philibert, D. C. Baldwin, Jr., and T. J. Nasca. "Causes of Death of Residents in Acgme-Accredited Programs 2000 through 2014: Implications for the Learning Environment." *Acad Med* 92, no. 7 (Jul 2017): 976-83.

Yao, Y., S. Zhao, X. Gao, Z. An, S. Wang, H. Li, Y. Li, *et al.* "General Self-Efficacy Modifies the Effect of Stress on Burnout in Nurses with Different Personality Types." *BMC Health Serv Res* 18, no. 1 (Aug 29 2018): 667.

Yoon, J. D., N. B. Hunt, K. C. Ravella, C. S. Jun, and F. A. Curlin. "Physician Burnout and the Calling to Care for the Dying: A National Survey." *Am J Hosp Palliat Care* 34, no. 10 (Dec 2017): 931-37.

Ziedelis, A. "Perceived Calling and Work Engagement among Nurses." *West J Nurs Res* 41, no. 6 (Jun 2019): 816-33.

Zulman, D. M., N. H. Shah, and A. Verghese. "Evolutionary Pressures on the Electronic Health Record: Caring for Complexity." *JAMA* 316, no. 9 (Sep 6 2016): 923-4.

ABOUT THE AUTHOR

Dr. Tianne Foster is a globally trained healthcare professional, researcher, and author committed to addressing the challenges of burnout. Originally from Calgary, Alberta, Canada, she earned her undergraduate degree in Cellular, Molecular, and Microbial Biology at the University of Calgary before pursuing medical training at the American University of the Caribbean, supported by an entrance scholarship. Her diverse medical education took her to the United Kingdom, United States, and Canada, providing invaluable insights into different healthcare systems.

With experience in administration, research, and clinical roles, Dr. Foster blends her expertise with interests and training in Conflict Management. She offers actionable solutions to promote well-being in individuals and organizations, as outlined in her book, Reality Check.

www.tiannefoster.com

TAKE YOUR JOURNEY FURTHER WITH THE REALITY CHECK WELLNESS WORKBOOK

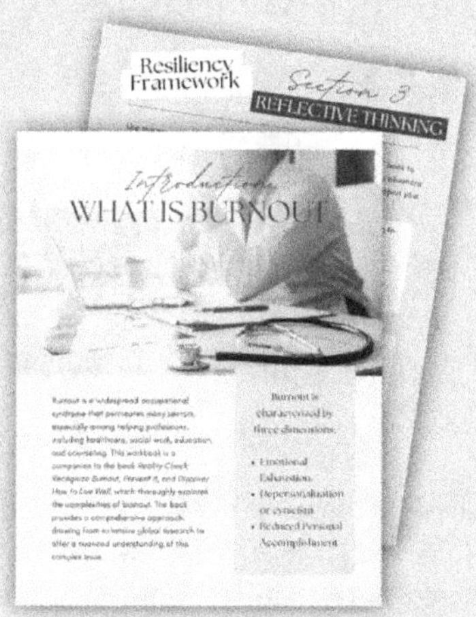

The Reality Check Wellness Workbook is your step-by-step guide to applying the principles from Reality Check in your daily life. Filled with reflection prompts, practical exercises, and actionable strategies, this workbook is designed to help you:

- **Build Self-Awareness:** Gain insight into your thoughts, behaviors, and habits.
- **Create Sustainable Well-Being:** Craft a plan for strength and balance in every aspect of your life.

Start your transformation today!

Learn more about the Reality Check Wellness Workbook at www.tiannefoster.com or scan the QR code to order directly.

DISCOVER THE SCIENCE-BACKED BENEFITS OF MINDFUL COLORING COMPANION

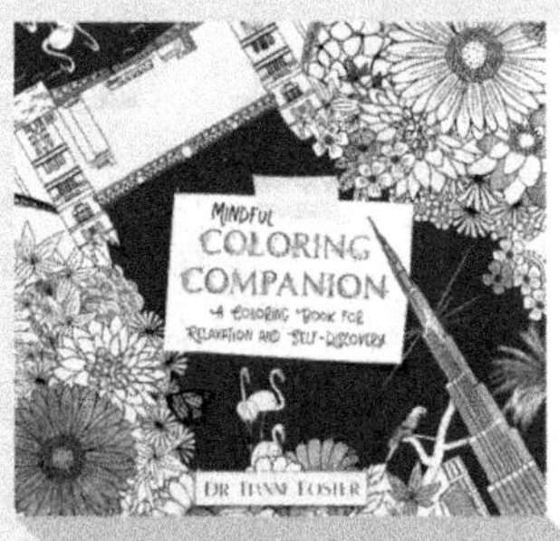

Coloring isn't just a pastime—it's supported by research as a way to reduce stress and encourage mindfulness, offering a reprieve from daily pressures. The Mindful Coloring Companion transforms creativity into a therapeutic experience, featuring breathtaking, photography-based designs of landscapes, iconic landmarks, and animals. This unique coloring book offers:

- **A Tool for Balance:** Cultivate emotional well-being through creative expression.
- **Self-Awareness Prompts:** Reflective prompts inspire deeper self-awareness and growth.
- **A Visual Journey:** Explore scenes from the author's travels around the world.

Make mindfulness part of your daily routine!

Explore the Mindful Coloring Companion at www.tiannefoster.com
or scan the QR code to purchase your copy.

TAILORED CONSULTATION FOR INDIVIDUALS AND ORGANIZATIONS

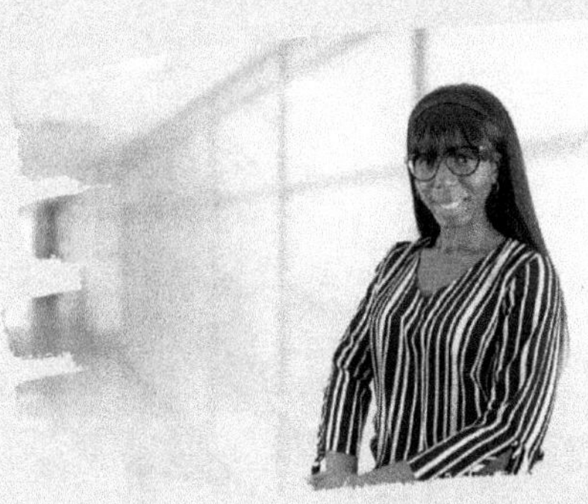

Dr. Tianne Foster offers expert consultation for individuals and businesses seeking to foster resilience, address workplace challenges, and enhance well-being. With a unique blend of experience across healthcare, research, and conflict management, her approach is tailored to meet the specific needs of each client.

Whether you're navigating burnout, improving team dynamics, or building a culture of wellness, Dr. Foster delivers insights and actionable solutions to help you thrive.

Learn more at www.tiannefoster.com and **schedule your consultation** by emailing booking@tiannefoster.com.

DYNAMIC SPEAKING ENGAGEMENTS TAILORED TO YOUR AUDIENCE

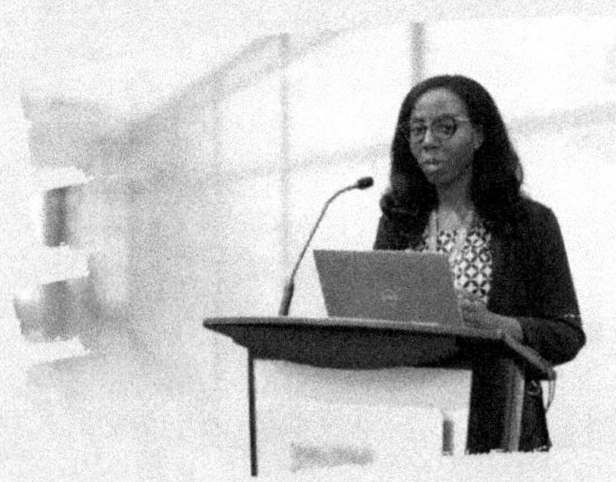

Dr. Tianne Foster is an inspirational speaker who engages audiences with impactful insights into wellness, resilience, and leadership. Drawing on her diverse expertise, she tailors every talk to align with the unique needs and interests of her audience.

Her speaking engagements are ideal for:

- Healthcare and corporate conferences.
- Team development workshops.
- Professional organizations seeking transformative discussions.

Learn more at www.tiannefoster.com and **schedule your event** by emailing booking@tiannefoster.com.

GROUP DISCUSSION GUIDE

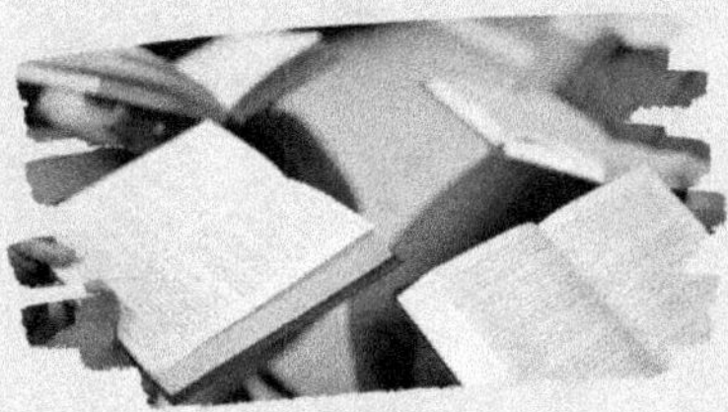

Reality Check opens the door to meaningful conversations about burnout, resilience, and well-being. Use this guide to spark insightful dialogue in any setting–teams, professional workshops, or casual gatherings.

Discussion Prompts:
- What key takeaways or moments resonated with you while reading Reality Check, and why?
- What are some practices in your team or workplace that effectively support well-being and reduce stress?
- What challenges do you or your group face when trying to maintain work-life balance, and how might these be addressed collectively?
- How does your group or workplace promote psychological safety and support mental health, and what steps could be taken to strengthen these efforts?
- Reflecting on Reality Check, what tools or strategies could your group use to strengthen workplace relationships and foster both inter- and intra-group collaboration?

Bulk Orders

Equip your team, organization, or community with the tools to combat burnout and build resilience. Bulk purchase discounts are available for groups, businesses, and educational institutions.
Learn more at https://www.tiannefoster.com/bulk-buy or email info@tiannefoster.com.

BE PART OF THE MOVEMENT

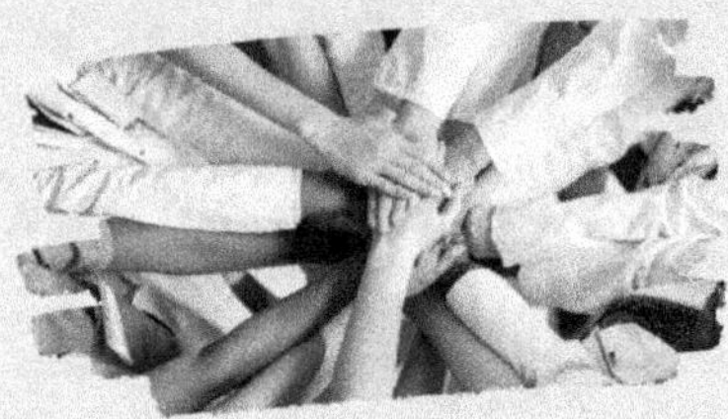

Thank you for joining me on this journey through Reality Check. Together, we can combat burnout and create thriving, engaging work environments.

Take the Next Steps:

1. Share Your Feedback:
Loved the book? Found it helpful? Please consider leaving a review on Amazon or Goodreads. Your feedback helps others find Reality Check and contributes to the conversation about meaningful change.

2. Discover More Tools:
Explore the Reality Check Wellness Workbook and Mindful Coloring Companion to enhance your experience. Visit www.tiannefoster.com for details.

3. Stay Connected:
Subscribe for exclusive updates and scan the QR code to find me on social media. You can also visit www.tiannefoster.com/contact.

4. Collaborate:
Interested in consultations, speaking engagements, or partnerships? Contact booking@tiannefoster.com.

Thank you for being part of this important conversation!